# Medical Problems
# in Pregnancy

D1795390

Dedicated to Mothers Everywhere

# Medical Problems in Pregnancy:
## their diagnosis and management

### John F. Mayberry
BSc, MD, BCh, MRCP
Clinical Teacher and Senior Registrar in Medicine,
University Hospital of Nottingham

### Andrew P. Bond
MD, BCh, MRCOG
Consultant in Obstetrics and Gynaecology,
Princess Margaret Hospital, Swindon and formerly Lecturer and
Senior Registrar in Obstetrics and Gynaecology, University of
Liverpool; Liverpool Maternity Hospital and Royal Liverpool
Hospital

### John S. Morris
MD, BCh, FRCP
Consultant Physician,
Bridgend General Hospital;
Clinical Teacher,
University Hospital of Wales, Cardiff and formerly Professor of
Medicine, University of Riyadh, Saudi Arabia

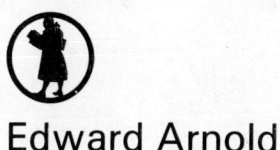

Edward Arnold

© John F. Mayberry, Andrew P. Bond and John S. Morris 1986

First published in Great Britain 1986 by
Edward Arnold (Publishers) Ltd,
41 Bedford Square,
London WC1B 3DQ

Edward Arnold (Australia) Pty Ltd,
80 Waverley Road,
Caulfield East,
Victoria 3145,
Australia

Edward Arnold,
3 East Read Street,
Baltimore,
Maryland 21202
USA

British Library Cataloguing in Publication Data

Mayberry, John F.
  Medical problems in pregnancy.
  1. Pregnancy, Complications of
  I. Title     II. Bond, Andrew P.
  III. Morris, John S.
  618.3     RG571

  ISBN 0-7131-4499-8

All Rights Reserved. No part of this publication may be
reproduced, stored in a retrieval system, or transmitted in any form
or by any means electronic, mechanical, photocopying, recording
or otherwise, without the prior permission of Edward Arnold
(Publishers) Ltd.

Whilst the advice and information in this book is believed to be
true and accurate at the date of going to press, neither the authors
nor the publisher can accept any legal responsibility or liability for
any errors or omissions that may be made.

Text set in 9/10 pt Times Compugraphic
by Colset Private Ltd, Singapore.
Printed and Bound in Great Britain by
Richard Clay (The Chaucer Press) Ltd, Bungay, Suffolk

# Preface

Pregnant women who are sick cause concern to both obstetricians and physicians. Although medical therapy during pregnancy is usually safe, the risks of teratogenesis are ever present. Initially this book was conceived as an integrated text dealing with a wide range of diseases and their management which may occur in pregnancy. This book is intended as a readily accessible source of up-to-date information for all concerned with the medical problems of pregnancy, including obstetricians, physicians, paediatricians and family doctors. It should also be of value to interested anaesthetists. The expectant mother demands an informed understanding of the particular complications that can arise during pregnancy and especially the effects of medical treatment.

Relationships between disease and pregnancy which may effect mother or child are the subjects of considerable research. Concern about possible teratogenic drug effects has limited the role of clinical trials and restricted the rapid introduction of new drugs. 'The old, the safe and the tried' has been a maxim that has guided many physicians and obstetricians in their joint management of obstetric medical problems. Whilst this philosophy is in the best interests of both mother and child, many recently introduced medical treatments have, as a result, found only a limited place in modern obstetric practice. In this book the available information on the safety of newer drugs in pregnancy is discussed. The early involvement of paediatricians is essential for the successful outcome of such pregnancies. Cooperation does not end at delivery and it is essential that combined care of mother and baby continues into the puerperium.

Medical complications during pregnancy can significantly alter the outlook for both mother and child; similarly pregnancy may worsen the prognosis of a disease that the mother had prior to conception. Pre-conceptual advice on the possibility of genetic traits appearing in future offspring is an important aspect of medical obstetric practice but the confines of space in a book of this size have not allowed us to explore this subject in detail. Some guidance on patient counselling is given but many decisions in this area are individual and this precludes a didactic approach.

We should like to thank Professor Barden and Harper and Row for permission to reproduce the tables on p. 81 and 84, Professor Friedman and John Wiley for permission to reproduce the table on p. 5, Dr. Lindheimer and the Journal of Reproductive Medicine for permission to reproduce the table on p. 3, Professor Montgomery and W.B. Saunders and Co. Ltd. to reproduce the table on p. 64 and Dr. West and Hospital Update for permission to reproduce the table on p. 82.

Our publishers, Edward Arnold, provided invaluable guidance in the final preparation of the manuscript. Finally we would like to thank our wives and children for their tolerance and encouragement.

1986                                                                                  JFM
                                                                                            APB
                                                                                            JSM

# Contents

# 1

# Hypertension and its management

Hypertension in pregnancy is one of the most important causes of maternal and perinatal morbidity and mortality. It occurs in about 1 per cent of all pregnancies and is a prominent cause of maternal death in England and Wales, usually because of cerebral haemorrhage.

The definition of hypertension and its treatment is controversial. The time-honoured diagnostic level of 140/90 mmHg or an increase of more than 20 mmHg in either the systolic or diastolic pressure are both of value, although arbitrary. Indeed, recent perinatal studies suggest that 140/90 mmHg represents the peak of maternal health rather than the beginning of disease.

## Blood pressure changes in pregnancy

Blood pressure varies during pregnancy. The systolic level falls initially to its lowest level during the second trimester, but rises again in the last trimester. The diastolic pressure is usually 10 mmHg below non-pregnant values until 30–32 weeks gestation. Changes in posture effect the recordings, higher values being recorded in the erect posture because of the compression of the aorta and inferior vena cava by the gravid uterus. This observation has been used as the basis of a clinical test described by Gant *et al* (1974).

## Hypertension in pregnancy

In 20 per cent of pregnant hypertensive patients, hypertension is present before pregnancy. The remaining 80 per cent are those who have pregnancy hypertension, formerly called toxaemia. If convulsions or coma supervene, the condition is termed eclampsia. Despite academic arguments concerning the definition of pregnancy hypertension, a working classification used by many, is a rise in systolic pressure of at least 30 mmHg or a rise in diastolic pressure of at least 15 mmHg over previously known blood pressure levels or a blood pressure of at least 140/90 mmHg on at least two occasions, 6 or more hours apart. Proteinuria indicates a count of more than 1 g/litre of protein in two random urine collections again taken more than 6 hours apart or more than 300 mg/litre of protein in a 24 hour urinary collection.

Because of the different aetiologies of pregnancy hypertension a classification is useful:

1. *Pregnancy associated hypertension (PAH) or pregnancy induced hypertension (PIH)*

   i. *Pre-eclampsia and eclampsia:* There may be hypertension, proteinuria, oedema and fits.
   ii. *Gestational hypertension:* There is hypertension during the pregnancy or for the first 10 days postpartum.

2. *Concurrent hypertension and pregnancy (CHP)*

   i. Acute hypertension of whatever aetiology but not due to the pregnancy.
   ii. Primary hypertension in pregnancy.
   iii. Secondary hypertension in pregnancy., eg. renal disease.

3. *Hypertensive tendency*

4. *Labile hypertension:* Temporary elevations of blood pressure which do not require treatment.

## Early detection of hypertension in pregnancy

It may be possible to detect women who will develop hypertension during their pregnancy using a technique described by Gant *et al* (1974). They found that 93 per cent of previously normotensive young women who became hypertensive in pregnancy had an elevation of their diastolic blood pressure of at least 20 mmHg within 5 minutes when turned from resting in the lateral recumbent position for 15 minutes to the supine position. This test was carried out between the 28th and 32nd weeks of gestation. Conversely 91 per cent of women who had no such rise in diastolic blood pressure did not become

**Table 1.1**   The roll over test (From Gant *et al*, 1974)

1. Performed during mid trimester
2. Patient rests in left lateral position for 15 minutes
3. Blood pressure is recorded
4. Patient rolls on to back
5. Blood pressure measured 1 and 5 minutes after rolling on to back
6. A rise of 20 mmHg is a positive test and implies that the patient will become hypertensive during the pregnancy

hypertensive during that pregnancy. Despite these findings this test has not gained wide acceptance.

## Classification of severity of hypertension in pregnancy

In addition to difficulties of definition, there is disagreement about the classification of its severity. Turner (1981) has divided hypertension into mild (nonproteinuric) pre-eclampsia and severe pre-eclampsia with proteinuria and an elevated blood pressure.

**Table 1.2** Classification of severity of hypertension in pregnant women (From Feitelson and Lyndheimer, 1972)

| Blood pressure | Mild | Moderate | Severe | Accelerated or malignant |
|---|---|---|---|---|
| Trimesters 1 and 2 | $\frac{130}{80}$ | $\frac{160}{100}$ | $\frac{180}{110}$ | |
| Trimester 3 | $\frac{140}{90}$ | $\frac{160}{110}$ | $\frac{180}{120}$ | |
| Proteinuria | 300 mg–1 g | 1–5 g | 5 g | |

## The clinical diagnosis of hypertension in pregnancy

The measurement of blood pressure is the subject of much discussion. For ease of reproduction the initial sound of systole is taken as the measure of systolic pressure. Muffling of sounds (Korotkov 4) rather than disappearance of sounds (Korotkov 5) is almost universally considered in obstetrics to be the best representation of diastolic pressure. Unless care is taken with the technique of measurement, it is very easy to obtain inaccurate figures and the following precautions must be observed:

1. The manometer must be accurate.
2. The arm must be at heart level.
3. Cuff size must be appropriate to the size of the arm.
4. The patient should be relaxed.

Examination of the patient's fundi allows direct inspection of the arteries and arterioles and the retinal changes that occur. These include arteriovenous nipping, flame-shaped haemorrhages, soft 'cotton-wool like' exudates and papilloedema. The more severe the hypertension the more likely the patient is to have haemorrhages, exudates and ultimately papilloedema.

## Effects of pregnancy hypertension on the fetus

The fetus of a hypertensive mother is at risk of intra-uterine growth retardation which can result in a mid trimester abortion. There is also risk of fetal distress or intra-uterine death in the third trimester. Placental abruption can occur. As a result of these risks the fetus often needs to be delivered prematurely. Intra-uterine growth retardation and death are particularly seen when chronic hypertension is associated with proteinuria (pre-eclampsia). The perinatal mortality of babies born to mothers with some form of hypertension is 25.4/1000 compared with 11.5/1000 among babies born to normotensive women.

**Table 1.3** Effects of maternal hypertension (Data from British Birth Survey, 1970)

|  | No. of women | No. of perinatal deaths | Perinatal mortality rate/1000 births |
|---|---|---|---|
| Normotensive | 10 787 | 207 | 19.2 |
| Concurrent Hypertension | 321 | 5 | 15.6 |
| Pre-eclampsia |  |  |  |
| 1.  Mild | 2 459 | 48 | 19.5 |
| 2.  Moderate | 610 | 11 | 18.1 |
| 3.  Severe | 830 | 28 | 33.7 |
| *Total* | 3 899 | 87 | 22.3 |
| Patients with concurrent hypertension who developed eclampsia | 163 | 5 | 30.7 |

There has been little change in perinatal mortality over the years, apart from the group with severe eclampsia. In the 1950s the perinatal mortality associated with this condition was 73.8/1000 total births, but by the 1970s had fallen to 33.7/1000 total births.

Friedman and Neff (1975) have analysed the significance of diastolic blood pressure and proteinuria without hypertension in relation to fetal survival in a study of almost 59 000 obstetric patients in the USA. Either measurement alone or in combination provide information about fetal risk.

In hypertensive women a raised plasma level of uric acid above 350 mmol/litre is associated with an increased perinatal mortality rate.

Hypertension is not associated with congenital abnormalities. It is associated, however, with a significant increase in respiratory complications after birth. Initial breathing difficulties and later, cyanotic attacks occur more frequently in the neonates of hypertensive mothers, possibly because of hypoxia during labour. For similar reasons convulsive episodes occur in the newborn.

**Table 1.4a** Stillbirth rates/1000 births for diastolic blood pressure by gestational age (Modified from Friedman and Neff, 1975)

| Diastolic pressure | Weeks of gestation | | | | |
| | 28–32 | 33–34 | 35–36 | 37 38 | 39–41 |
| --- | --- | --- | --- | --- | --- |
| 65–74 | 7 | 6 | 4 | 5 | 5 |
| 75–84 | 8 | 6 | 6 | 4 | 3 |
| 85–94 | 9 | 8 | 6 | 5 | 5 |
| > 95 | 21 | 19 | 16 | 9 | 9 |

**Table 1.4b** Stillbirth rates/1000 births for proteinuria without hypertension by gestational age

| Proteinuria | Weeks of gestation | | | | |
| | 28–32 | 33–34 | 35–36 | 37–38 | 39–41 |
| --- | --- | --- | --- | --- | --- |
| None | 10 | 8 | 6 | 5 | 4 |
| Trace | 11 | 11 | 10 | 8 | 10 |
| + | 6 | 10 | 16 | 11 | 6 |
| + + | 40 | 44 | 17 | 25 | 41 |
| + + + | 58 | 56 | 24 | 19 | 22 |

Whether treatment of maternal hypertension is of benefit to the fetus remains uncertain. Two controlled trials of antihypertensive treatment of pregnant women indicate a reduction in the number of mid trimester abortions amongst those treated.

## Effects of pregnancy hypertension on the mother

Severe hypertension carries with it a significant risk of cerebral haemorrhage, although this risk is no different from that of male hypertensives. The particular risk, however, is the development of pre-eclampsia which is unique to pregnancy and is characterized by hypertension, oedema and proteinuria. Eclampsia, the sequel to untreated or mismanaged pre-eclampsia, is a convulsive state also specific to pregnancy and the immediate puerperium. The convulsions resemble grand mal epileptic fits. The condition rarely occurs before the third trimester and may or may not be associated with previous hypertension. The signs of pre-eclampsia include, elevation of blood pressure beyond 140/90 mmHg on two separate occasions 24 hours apart or a rise in blood pressure of 20 mmHg over the first trimester recordings associated with proteinuria of at least 0.5 g/litre in 24 hours. Oedema may or may not occur. Renal function may be impaired and should be monitored with a fluid chart, recording daily output together with specific gravity or osmolality of the urine.

Reduced urinary output and inability to concentrate the urine indicate impaired renal function. The blood urea is usually lower in pregnancy so values acceptable as normal outside pregnancy may indicate a deterioration in renal function during pregnancy.

The recurrence of pre-eclampsia in a subsequent pregnancy is unusual and long-term complications are unlikely. If hypertension or renal damage persist an underlying disease is present. The only continuing factor seems to be an hereditary predisposition to pre-eclampsia in the daughters of women who have had the disorder.

## Treatment

Labile hypertension is not associated with fetal or maternal problems and consequently it is essential to establish the diagnosis of pregnancy associated hypertension before treatment is started. A raised blood pressure in the antenatal clinic is only an index of suspicion. Arrangements must be made to assess blood pressure and fetal well-being for a period of 3 days. The basal blood pressure, as taken first thing in the morning, with the patient in bed, is the best prognostic indicator. If this continues to be raised for more than 24 hours the diagnosis is established and treatment should be instituted.

### Bed-rest

Bed-rest has been recommended for patients with pregnancy hypertension to control blood pressure and oedema and to increase urine output and plancental blood flow. However, its necessity is now largely questioned and it is apparently no more effective than ambulatory management in preventing proteinuria, serious hypertension or eclampsia. When 346 nulliparous patients with pregnancy induced hypertension were admitted to hospital by Hauth *et al* (1976) and allowed to walk about freely 85 per cent became normotensive within 5 days and only 6 per cent needed to be delivered within 7 days. In addition, it is doubtful whether placental perfusion is diminished by exercise and certainly human placental lactogen values are not raised by bed-rest in either normal or abnormal pregnancies. When strict bed-rest has been abandoned in favour of more ambulant regimens in the management of hypertensive patients, the perinatal mortality rate has improved. Bed-rest during the antenatal period theoretically increases the risk of maternal death from pulmonary embolism. Mild hypertensives can consequently be managed at home, but patients with diastolic blood pressures in excess of 105 mmHg, or proteinuria or other evidence of fetal compromise require hospital admission.

### Sedation

Blood pressure falls during sleep in both normotensive and hypertensive subjects, although this may not be true in pre-eclampsia. As a result, sedation was, at one time, a popular treatment of pregnancy hypertension. Controlled trials, however, do not indicate a useful effect of sedation in pregnancy hypertension and it may even endanger the fetus as a result of withdrawal effects, feeding difficulties and disturbed mother–child bonding.

## Drug treatment

The aims of hypotensive therapy in pregnant women are protection of the mother from the effects of high blood pressure, especially cerebral haemorrhage. Control of blood pressure until fetal maturity is achieved minimises the dangers of prematurity. Maintenance of uteroplacental perfusion encourages normal intra-uterine fetal growth and avoids hypoxia.

### Central sympathetic inhibitors

*Methyldopa* Methyl noradrenaline is the active metabolite of methyldopa which produces the antihypertensive effect. It reduces blood pressure in concomitant or essential hypertensives at a dose of 0.5–4.0 g/day in 90 per cent of cases. Its use is limited in about 12 per cent of women because of side effects including drowsiness, depression, orthostatic hypotension, nausea, diarrhoea and Coomb's positive haemolytic anaemia. Until recently, it has been the drug of choice for control of hypertension during pregnancy and probably has been used more frequently than others. Although it crosses the placental barrier and appears in breast milk, no obvious teratogenic effects have been reported; although, at birth, head circumference is reduced in the offspring of patients treated between 16 and 20 weeks gestation. The effect does not seem to be permanent and there is no subsequent intellectual impairment. It is, therefore, a safe and helpful drug in the management of pregnancy associated hypertension.

*Diuretics* Diuretics are first-line agents in the treatment of essential hypertension, but they are best avoided in pregnancy for several reasons and are completely ineffective in severe pre-eclampsia. They may result in electrolyte derangement, including neonatal hyponatraemia, reduced placental steroidogenesis and neonatal thrombocytopaenia.

*Vasodilators* Hydralazine relaxes arteriolar muscle and decreases peripheral resistance thereby reducing blood pressure. The baroreceptor reflex is unaffected so the fall in blood pressure results in tachycardia and an increase in the cardiac output. There is an increase in cerebral, renal and placental blood flow. However, if the fall in blood pressure exceeds 15 per cent placental perfusion is reduced.

Oral hydralazine alone, reduces blood pressure in about 50 per cent of pregnancy associated hypertensives, but if it is combined with a $\beta$ blocker such as propranolol the effect is greatly enhanced. Provided the daily dose of hydralazine does not exceed 150 mg and the daily dose of propranolol 240 mg, no adverse fetal effects are seen. It may be advisable to withdraw the $\beta$ blocker prior to labour.

Hydralazine is of particular value in the control of acute hypertension in pregnant women, but all parenteral routes of administration have problems:

1. *Intramuscular.* A proportion of patients have an exaggerated response to the drug as they are genetically unable to metabolize it or have impaired renal excretion.
2. *Intravenous bolus.* This can cause sudden abrupt hypotension and can also produce side effects which may mimic eclampsia.
3. *Slow intravenous infusion.* This route is preferable although it is associated with the above side effects. The suggested rate of infusion is 2–5 mg/hour by an infusion pump, which allows careful regulation of the dose. This regimen is particularly useful in fulminant pre-eclamptic toxaemia and eclampsia.

Doses in excess of 200 mg of hydralazine a day have been associated with a systemic lupus erythematosus-like syndrome, but this has not yet been reported in pregnancy.

*Care must be taken if the patient has an epidural block as this will act synergistically with hydralazine to produce a dramatic and potentially dangerous drop in blood pressure.* Prior to epidural blockade, antihypertensive therapy should be considerably reduced.

### Adrenoreceptor blockade

$\beta$ blockers are probably amongst the most commonly used antihypertensives in the non-pregnant population. Their role in pregnancy is currently being assessed. There are three main groups of interest:

1. Non-specific $\beta$ blockers such as propranolol and oxprenolol.
2. $\beta_1$ specific blockers such as metoprolol.
3. Combined $\alpha$ and $\beta_1$ blockers and $\beta_2$ agonists such as labetalol.

*Non-specific $\beta$ blockers*  Propranolol has no acute hypotensive action when given parenterally and usually requires 2 weeks or more of oral administration to lower blood pressure in the non-pregnant woman. It produces a fall in cardiac output and generalized vasoconstriction. Non-specific $\beta$ blockers also promote myometrial contraction and lead to neonatal hypoglycaemia, bradycardia and respiratory depression, particularly when the placenta is small and the baby immature. Until recently, such drugs have not been recommended for the management of hypertension in pregnancy. If hypertension develops in the puerperium, it is important to remember that propranolol is excreted in breast milk and breast-fed babies could develop bradycardia and respiratory distress.

$\beta$ blockade for hypertension in pregnancy seems to confer benefits on the fetus. $\beta$ blocking agents reduce fetal morbidity when compared with methyldopa and hydralazine. Early anecdotal reports of a high incidence of fetal death have not been substantiated in larger controlled studies, although questions remain as to intra-uterine growth retardation, neonatal bradycardia and hypotension and neonatal hypoglycaemia.

*$\beta_1$ specific blockers* Insufficient work on the safety and efficacy of such agents as metoprolol limit their use in pregnancy. Because of cardioselectivity they are less likely to be associated with intra-uterine growth retardation (Sandstrom, 1978).

*Combined $\alpha$, $\beta_1$ blocker and $\beta_2$ agonist (labetalol)* This drug causes peripheral vasodilatation without affecting the cardiac output. It rapidly reduces blood pressure at doses of 400–800 mg a day, but does not reduce placenta blood flow. It both crosses the placenta and appears in breast milk.

*Calcium antagonists*
The role of nifedepine in the treatment of pregnancy associated hypertension is currently under assessment. Preliminary results suggest that it is likely to become an important option in treatment.

*Diazoxide*
This drug no longer has a place in the treatment of hypertension. It causes hyperglycaemia and may induce alopecia in the fetus.

# Management of hypertensive problems in pregnancy
## Established hypertension

Two major questions are whether the pregnancy should be terminated or whether antihypertensive agents should be changed. Termination seems indicated when a stroke, myocardial infarction or heart failure have previously occurred. Although few antihypertensive drugs are teratogenic many have undesirable side-effects in late pregnancy and it is probably wise to change to one of the agents commonly used during pregnancy. This is particularly true of the diuretic $\beta$ blocker combination on which many patients are controlled. Consideration should be given to the use of methyldopa, hydralazine and propranolol or labetalol.

## Hypertension arising in pregnancy
### With a mature fetus

When hypertension develops after the 37th week of gestation early delivery is appropriate.

### With an immature fetus

In this group of patients if the hypertension is moderate they should receive treatment with antihypertensive drugs and the drugs of choice at present are methyldopa, labetalol or a combination of hydralazine and propranolol. In severe hypertension with pre-eclampsia, eclampsia, fetal growth retardation or fetal distress, delivery is indicated regardless of gestational age.

**Table 1.5** Indications for delivery of hypertensive patients regardless of gestational age

| Severe pre-eclampsia | 1. | Blood pressure greater than 160/110 *or* |
|---|---|---|
| | 2. | Oliguria (less than 600 ml of urine in 24 hours) *or* |
| | 3. | Cyanosis or pulmonary oedema *or* |
| | 4. | Marked proteinuria (more than 5 g in 24 hours) |
| Fetal growth retardation | 1. | Ultrasonic monitoring of fetal thoracic and biparietal diameters fall below normal range |
| Fetal distress | 1. | Positive oxytocin challenge test (25–50% false positives). Caution must be used in interpreting this sign as an indication of impending fetal death *or* |
| | 2. | A positive non-stress test *or* |
| | 3. | Meconium stained amniotic fluid |

If intensive care facilities are available, prolongation of pregnancy until the fetus becomes viable is possible. Management should include prevention of convulsions with low dose diazepam or chlormethiazole. In the USA parenteral magnesium sulphate is often given. A loading dose of 10 g magnesium sulpate is given as a 50 per cent solution intramuscularly; or alternatively, 4 mg is given intravenously as a 20 per cent solution over 5 minutes. Therapeutic levels are achieved when the concentration of magnesium in the blood is between 5.5 and 9 mg/litre. Toxic effects appear at 12 mg/litre when patellar reflexes disappear and the respiratory rate falls below 16 breaths/minute. As the drug is exclusively cleared by the kidneys, urine output must be carefully monitored.

Further aspects of this form of intensive treatment should include automatic monitoring of blood pressure. Normotensive values may also be obtained by administration of 20 mg of intravenous hydralazine followed by a slow infusion (40 mg of hydralazine in 500 ml of 5 per cent dextrose) or 20 mg of labetalol as an infusion every hour. The dose can be doubled every 30 minutes until an adequate reduction in blood pressure has been obtained or a dosage of 160 mg/hour is reached.

Diuretics or steroids may be necessary to reduce cerebral oedema.

There should be cardiotographic monitoring of the fetus and fetal distress is an indication for delivery.

The maternal clotting profile is monitored every 4–6 hours and a deterioration in renal function is also an indication that the pregnancy should be terminated.

If pre-eclampsia fails to improve within 24–48 hours of medical management elective delivery is mandatory. Sedation and hypotensive therapy should be continued for at least 48 hours postpartum to prevent recurrence of eclampsia. After, the condition usually settles rapidly with a marked diuresis. If the fetus dies *in utero* the condition also subsides rapidly.

## Further reading

Rubin, P.C. (1981). Beta blockers in pregnancy. *New England Journal of Medicine* **305**, 1323.

Stirrat, G.M. (1981). Management of hypertension in pregnancy. *British Journal of Hospital Medicine* **26**, 135.

## References

Alvarez, R.R. (1978). Pre-eclampsia and renal diseases in pregnancy. *Clinical Obstetrics and Gynaecology* **21**, 881.

Chamberlain, G., Philipp, E., Howlett, B. and Masters, K. (1978). British Births, 1970. In *Volume 2 Obstetric Care*. Heinemann, London.

Feitelson, P.J. and Lindheimer, M.D. (1972). Management of hypertensive gravidas. *Journal of Reproductive Medicine* **8**, 111.

Freidman, E.A. and Neff, R.K. (1975). *Hypertension in Pregnancy*. Edited by Lindheimer, M., Katz, A. and Zuspan, F. John Wiley, London.

Gant, N.F., Chand, S., Worley, R.J., Whalley, P.J., Crosby, C.D. and MacDonald, P.C. (1974). A clinical test useful for predicting the development of acute hypertension in pregnancy. *American Journal of Obstetrics and Gynecology* **120**, 1.

Gant, N.F., Worley, R.J., Cunningham, F.G., and Whalley, P.J. (1978). Clinical management of pregnancy-induced hypertension. *Clinical Obstetrics and Gynecology* **21**, pp. 397–409.

Hauth, J.C., Cunningham, F.G. and Whalley, P.J. (1976). Management of pregnancy-induced hypertension in the nullipara. *Obstetrics and Gynecology* **48**, 253.

Matthews, D.D., Shuttleworth, T.P. and Hamilton, E.F.B. (1978). Modern trends in management of non-albuminuric hypertension in late pregnancy. *British Medical Journal* **2**, 623.

Sandstrom, B. (1978). Antihypertensive treatment with the adrenergic beta receptor blocker metoprolol during pregnancy. *Gynecology and Obstetric Investigation* **9**, 195.

Turner, G.M. (1981). Management of pre-eclampsia and eclampsia. *British Journal of Hospital Medicine* **26**, 120.

# 2

# Venous thrombosis and its management

This chapter is divided into two sections—the first dealing with venous thrombosis and its treatment during pregnancy and the second with the use of anticoagulant drugs.

## Venous thrombosis

When superficial and deep vein thrombosis (DVT) and pulmonary embolism are considered together, an acute episode complicates 1 in 70 pregnancies. The death rate from pulmonary embolism during the years 1976 to 1978 was 26/million maternities and 70/million following a Caesarian section in England and Wales.

**Table 2.1** Risk factors for thromboembolism in pregnancy

---

1. Increased age (especially over 30) and parity (fourth or subsequent child).
2. Excessive obesity (over 76 kg)
3. Prolonged bed-rest
4. Caesarian section leads to a ten-fold increase in incidence
5. Suppressed lactation due to oestrogen administration
6. Previous history of thromboembolism
7. Sickle cell anaemia and anaemia in general
8. Congestive cardiac failure
9. Dehydration
10. Shock
11. Puerperal sepsis

   Most thrombotic events occur postpartum

---

The diagnosis of deep vein thrombosis is suggested by complaints of calf pain and physical signs such as tenderness in the calf, unilateral oedema and increased skin temperature. There should be a difference of 2 cm or more in the measurement of calf circumferences.

Pulmonary embolism can be silent or cause sudden death usually due to a cardiac arrest. However, the classical signs are sudden collapse, chest pain and air hunger. The patient is cyanosed, breathless and has a raised jugular venous pressure (JVP).

Haemoptysis, pleural pain and a friction rub are usually associated with a smaller embolism and pulmonary infarction.

## Investigation

### Doppler ultrasonic scanning

This is a useful screening method for the diagnosis of deep vein thrombosis in pregnancy. The ultrasonic probe is placed over the femoral vein, which is medial to the artery. Distorted flow patterns and the absence of flow are easily identified. There is a characteristic rushing sound if the calf is gently compressed. A similar response results from respiration or the Valsalva manoeuvre. Due to the presence of collateral venous channels in the calf, ultrasound does not detect minor calf vein thrombosis. The advantages of ultra-sonography are that it is not invasive and can be performed with small portable units which may be used at the bedside. Compared with phlebography, ultrasonography has an accuracy of 85–95 per cent in the detection of major vein thrombosis.

### Limb impedance plethysmography

The calf veins are allowed to fill under resting conditions with a pressure cuff inflated for 45 seconds or, if necessary, 3 minutes. Resistance electrodes are placed under the cuff, which is then released rapidly and the rate of emptying of the venous channels is recorded to detect obstruction to venous flow. During the second half of pregnancy the gravid uterus affects the pattern of venous flow and the method is only 50 per cent accurate in detecting calf vein thrombosis.

### Pulse volume recording

A cuff is used instead of strain gauges. It measures the venous outflow because a known amount of pressure is applied to the calf cuffs. Response to compression and respiration identifies venous occlusion. The major disadvantage is a false positive result, although this is rare. Ten per cent investigations may be falsely negative.

### Ascending phlebography

In skilled hands this is undoubtedly the most accurate method of investigation. It has the added advantage that it indicates the adherence of the thrombus to the vein wall. Where a DVT is present 95 per cent are accurately detected. However, it tends to be avoided in pregnancy because of the radiation hazard to the fetus; although some protection may be given by shielding the mother's abdomen with a lead apron. Where the diagnosis is in great doubt this procedure should be undertaken for the risk of needless anticoagulation is considerable.

### Isotope venography and lung scanning

Microspheres of albumin or fibrin micro-aggregates labelled with $^{99}Tc^m$ (technetium) appears to be a safe and accurate method for the diagnosis of thrombosis during pregnancy. The agent has a short half-life of about 6 hours and the dose required is small; most material is retained in the lungs and little crosses the placenta. The flow of radio-active particles in the deep veins is recorded with a gamma camera and macro-aggregates congregate around an occluding thrombus resulting in a 'hot spot'. This method detects 85–98 per cent of iliofemoral thrombosis; but false positive findings are frequent. A major advantage is the detection of pulmonary emboli on lung scanning with only one injection.

### Electrocardiographic changes associated with a pulmonary embolus

These are transitory and may only last a few hours. They include right axis deviation, right bundle branch block, prominent S waves in Standard lead I, Q waves and inverted T waves in Standard lead III, p pulmonale and there may also be right ventricular hypertrophy if there have been recurrent emboli. The T waves in $V_1$ and $V_3$ are inverted and may resemble a myocardial infarction pattern.

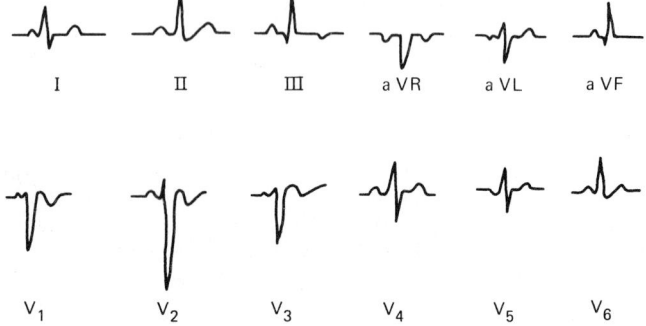

**Fig. 2.1**   ECG changes of an acute pulmonary embolus. An S wave appears in lead I and a Q wave in lead III, T wave inversion in III and over the right ventricle and incomplete right bundle branch block. The changes may be slight and easily overlooked.

## Treatment

Pregnancy itself produces changes in the coagulation profile.

**Table 2.2** Effects of pregnancy on coagulation (Modified from Laros and Alger, 1979)

| Factor/Activity | Effects of pregnancy |
|---|---|
| 1. Platelets | i. Slow decrease during pregnancy |
| | ii. Further fall after delivery |
| | iii. Increase 3rd–5th day after postpartum |
| 2. Fibrinogen | i. Increased during antenatal period |
| | ii. Prompt fall after delivery |
| 3. Factor V | i. Immediate increase after delivery |
| 4. Factors VII, IX and X | i. Increased throughout pregnancy |
| | ii. Gradual decrease in puerperium |
| 5. Factor VIII | i. Progressive increase during pregnancy |
| | ii. Although there is an immediate decrease after delivery, it is followed by an increase |
| 6. Factor XI and XIII | i. Decreased during pregnancy |
| | ii. Return to normal in puerperium |
| 7. Fibrin degradation products | i. Increased during labour and postpartum |
| 8. Fibrinolysis | i. Decreased during 2nd and 3rd trimesters |
| | ii. Return to normal after delivery |

## Use of heparin

Heparin does not cross the placenta and from the fetal aspect it is the safest anticoagulant to use during pregnancy. Unfortunately it must be given parenterally, but this can be self-administered subcutaneously and it is feasible to use this method throughout pregnancy and the puerperium.

## Antithrombotic therapy in pregnancy

Villasanta (1965) reviewed 163 cases of antepartum thromboembolic disease that were not treated with anticoagulants and found that 26 (16 per cent) had pulmonary emboli and there were 21 (13 per cent) deaths. In 134 cases of antepartum thromboembolic disease in which anticoagulants were used the incidence of thromboembolism was similar (19 per cent) but there was only one maternal death (1 per cent).

Five to ten thousand units of heparin are given as an intravenous bolus injection, followed by 1000 to 1200 units/hour as an infusion. Heparin should not be mixed in dextrose as this reduces its activity. A small portable infusion pump is the best mechanism for administration of the heparin and produces less episodes of bleeding than intermittent bolus injections.

The effect of heparin can be monitored in various ways which include:

1. Activated partial thromboplastin time (aPTT).
2. Lee–White clotting time (LWCT).
3. Activated clotting time (ACT).
4. Thrombin clotting time (TCT).

aPTT is a more sensitive and accurate test than the LWCT, but there is evidence that aPTTs greater than 70 seconds are poorly reproducible and hence unreliable when assessing higher degrees of anticoagulation. The ACT is a rapid, more precise, whole blood clotting time than the LWCT and is very useful in monitoring therapy. Its disadvantage is that it must be performed at the bedside. The thrombin clotting time is easy to perform and accurate. Usually only one of these techniques is available in an individual laboratory. The role of anticoagulation is to increase the value of the TCT to 2.5 times control, whole blood clotting time to 1.5 times control, ACT to twice control and aPTT to 2.5 to 3 times control readings.

Intravenous heparin should be given for 48 hours. Anticoagulation with warfarin may be undertaken in the puerperium. During pregnancy, oral anticoagulants are ideally avoided and either subcutaneous or intravenous heparin should be used long-term. However, many patients are unable to comply with such a regime for the whole of their pregnancies. A reasonable compromise is to cover the first trimester with heparin, then to use oral anticoagulants until the 36th week, after which heparin should be again used.

**Administration of subcutaneous heparin**

The concentrated 25 000 i.u of heparin in 1 ml should be used with a diabetic syringe and a 25 or 26 gauge needle. A fold of skin is gently raised on the outer aspect of the abdominal wall, the skin cleansed and the needle inserted to a depth of 1 cm at right angles to the skin and the exact dose of heparin injected. The needle is carefully withdrawn. *The injection site is not massaged.* Arms and legs are best avoided as injection sites. Local haematoma formation can be reduced by local application of ice prior to injection and sites should be altered with each injection.

**Long-term heparin: its regulation and management**

Sodium heparin is cheaper and has a longer duration of action than calcium heparin. Up to 10 000 units every 12 hours may be required. Plasma levels will need to be monitored weekly and should be checked 2 to 4 hours after the subcutaneous injection when serum levels are at their peak. A plasma level of 0.02 to 0.3 i.u./ml provides effective protection against thrombosis in pregnancy.

At the beginning of labour, heparin can be temporarily discontinued or reduced to 5 000 i.u every 12 hours. Spinal anaesthesia should be avoided because of the risk of local bleeding. A similar dose is used in the puerperium for 5 or 6 weeks after delivery to prevent extension of the original thrombosis.

## The value of prophylactic anticoagulation

If a patient has had previous thromboembolism she will be at risk of recurrence. Prophylactic treatment should begin 4–6 weeks before the gestation time at which the previous episode occurred. Where the thromboembolism is unrelated to pregnancy the greatest risk time is the puerperium and prophylaxis should be given for 4–6 weeks after delivery and also in late pregnancy if there are additional risk factors such as obesity or prolonged bed-rest.

A regime which may be followed is 5 000 i.u subcutaneously every 8 to 12 hours. The TCT is only minimally elevated and monitoring is unnecessary. Dextran 70 appears to prevent pulmonary emboli but not thrombosis in the legs. When given prophylactically during labour or Caesarian section it is likely to reduce the incidence of pulmonary embolism. It can be used safely with epidural anaesthesia but should be avoided if there is cardiac or renal failure.

## Side-effects and contraindications to heparin therapy

**Table 2.3** Heparin therapy: side-effects and contraindications

*Side-effects of heparin therapy*

| | | |
|---|---|---|
| 1. | Haemorrhage: | This is seen in about 4% of patients where the blood levels exceed 0.5 units of heparin/ml |
| 2. | Osteoporosis: | This may occur if given in doses greater than 15 000 i.u/day for 6 months. This is rare in pregnancy but may be prevented by giving 12 g of calcium gluconate daily |
| 3. | Hypotension | |
| 4. | Alopecia | |
| 5. | Allergic reactions | |
| 6. | Thrombocytopaenia | |

*Contraindications to heparin therapy*

1. Threatened abortion
2. Significant risk of intracranial haemorrhage eg. in eclampsia

## Oral anticoagulants

Subcutaneous heparin is safe and effective, whereas oral anticoagulants are associated with teratogenicity. However, a number of women with artificial cardiac valves on long-term anticoagulants have had successful pregnancies.

## Teratogenic effects of warfarin and other coumarin anticoagulants

Warfarin is a small molecule which is loosely bound to albumin and easily crosses the placenta. During the first trimester, especially the fourth to eighth weeks, it may cause abnormalities of nasal cartilages, bone epiphyses and brachydactyly. In the USA, problems later in pregnancy have been attributed to fetal haemorrhage but this may reflect the more widespread used of bishydroxycoumarin which is a slow acting cumulative agent.

### Management of anticoagulation in the pregnant patient with a valve replacement

When considering the continued use of anticoagulants the risk to the fetus has to be balanced against the risk of stopping therapy to the mother. There is a real risk of thromboembolism in patients with prosthetic valves, when anticoagulants are stopped or interrupted, though this is less with newer cloth-covered valves. The risk is greater with mitral than aortic valve replacements, but anticoagulation should be continued in both cases. Anticoagulants are seldom needed if a tissue valve replacement is used and the advantages of a biological valve in a young woman who may wish to have a family are obvious although they show less durability than artificial valves.

An alternative to oral anticoagulants is heparin therapy throughout pregnancy or to use it during the first trimester and again shortly before term. The difficulty lies in predicting the date of conception.

# Further reading

Bonnar, J. (1981). Venous thromboembolism and pregnancy. *Clinics in Obstetrics and Gynaecology* **8**, 455.

Howie, P.W. (1977). Thromboembolism. *Clinics in Obstetrics and Gynaecology* **4**, 397.

Laros, R.K. and Alger, L.S. (1979). Thromboembolism and pregnancy. *Clinical Obstetrics and Gynecology* **22**, 871.

Moseley, P. and Kerstein, M.D. (1980). Pregnancy and thrombophlebitis. *Surgery, Gynecology and Obstetrics* **150**, 593.

Oakley, C. and Doherty, P. (1976). Pregnancy in patients after valve replacement. *British Heart Journal* **38**, 1140.

Redman, C.W.G. (1979). Coagulation problems in human pregnancy. *Postgraduate Medical Journal* **55**, 367.

# 3

# Heart disease in pregnancy

Cardiac problems in pregnant women usually predate the onset of pregnancy. The quality of management and the course of the disease before pregnancy have an important bearing on what happens during the antenatal period. In the Western world congenital heart disease in pregnant women is now as frequent as rheumatic valvular disease, while in poorer countries and immigrant communities rheumatic heart disease remains prominent.

## Circulatory adjustments during pregnancy

The main changes include an alteration in cardiac output and circulating blood volume. There is a minimal increase in heart rate, increased cardiac output is achieved by an increased stroke volume. The response to *exercise* changes during pregnancy and here an increase in cardiac output is achieved by an increase in heart rate rather than stroke volume. At one time it was believed that cardiac output fell at the end of pregnancy. This fall is, however, only apparent and is due to compression of the inferior vena cava which impedes venous return in the supine position. In a few patients a

**Table 3.1** Summary of physiological changes in pregnancy

| | | |
|---|---|---|
| *Cardiac output* | 1. | Increases from end of first trimester to a maximum at 20th week of gestation |
| | 2. | Maintained at a level of 130–140 % throughout pregnancy |
| | 3. | Stroke volume and heart rate are raised |
| | 4. | *Maximal load is not at 36 weeks gestation as used to be thought* |
| *Blood pressure* | 1. | Small fall in systolic pressure |
| | 2. | Greater fall in diastolic pressure |
| | 3. | Pulse pressure (Systolic — diastolic) increased |
| *Oedema* | 1. | More marked with increased gestation |
| *Postpartum changes* | 1. | Blood volume is increased and this may precipitate heart failure in patients with structural heart disease |

**Table 3.2**  Summary of physical signs that occur in a normal pregancy

| | | |
|---|---|---|
| *Pulse* | 1. | Full and may be collapsing |
| | 2. | Capillary pulsation |
| *Pulse pressure* | 1. | Increased |
| *Apex beat* | 1. | Displaced outwards |
| *Triple rhythm* | 1. | Present |
| *Murmurs* | 1. | Short mid systolic ejection murmur |
| | 2. | Best heard at apex and/or in pulmonary area |
| | 3. | Systolic extracardiac murmurs occur in about 15 % of pregnant women. These may continue into diastole and are best heard at the left sternal border |

**Table 3.3**  Normal electrocardiographic changes in pregnancy

1. Axis shifts to left
2. In some patients a Q wave will persist in lead III until after delivery. This becomes less deep on inspiration
3. The T wave in lead III is often inverted but will become upright on inspiration
4. ST segment changes and T wave changes similar to those seen in ischaemic heart disease may occur
5. Atrial and ventricular extrasystoles are common
6. Bouts of supraventricular tachycardia may occur

parasympathetic response occurs resulting in bradycardia but no rise in peripheral resistance and syncope may result. (*Supine hypotensive syndrome*). This is most evident in polyhydramnios or multiple pregnancy.

# Heart disease in pregnancy

The hyperkinetic circulation of pregnancy accentuates cardiac murmurs associated with stenotic valvular disease. Mitral stenosis, for example, may be clearly heard in pregnancy and less obvious in the puerperium. By contrast, many patients whose hearts are normal are suspected of cardiac disease in the course of pregnancy and it may be difficult to be certain whether structural heart disease is present or not. Such patients should receive careful antenatal supervision followed by full investigation after childbirth.

Grading of symptoms is unhelpful in assessing outcome in pregnancy (Szekely and Turner, 1968). However, regular supervision of the patient with organic heart disease is required to detect pulmonary oedema or arrhythmias. General principles include the prompt treatment of respiratory infections and anaemia. Signs of pulmonary oedema should be treated with complete bed-rest in hospital, preferably on a cardiac bed to reduce intrathoracic blood volume. Diuretics and digoxin may be required, or even surgery.

Termination is not an option for the treatment of cardiac failure as it carries an equal risk to that of continuing with the pregnancy.

Vaginal delivery with the use of forceps to shorten the second stage is the aim. Caesarian section should be elective and not follow any sort of 'trial of labour.'

# Rheumatic heart disease

## Acute rheumatic fever

The major manifestations of acute rheumatic fever are carditis, polyarthritis, chorea, erythema marginatum and subcutaneous nodules. Minor manifestations include arthralgia and fever. On investigation there may be prolongation of the P–R interval and elevation of the ESR or C–reactive protein. A combination of two major, or one major and two or more minor manifestations is sufficient to establish the diagnosis, particularly if there is evidence of a preceding streptococcal infection.

Chorea is more common in women under 25 years old and when it occurs during pregnancy is termed chorea gravidarum. Such women have usually had chorea previously and many have rheumatic valvular disease.

There is no evidence that pregnancy predisposes to recurrence of polyarthritis or carditis and it is debatable whether pregnancy increases the tendency to recurrence of chorea. Acute carditis and pregnancy is, however, a serious association. Several fatal cases have been reported in whom pre-existing valve lesions were absent. A number of patients died suddenly in labour or after delivery.

### Investigation

The ESR and C–reactive protein are almost always increased during the course of active rheumatic fever. The antistreptolysin titre exceeds 250 Todd units, reaching a peak about 3 weeks later and returns to normal in 2–4 months. Throat cultures are positive in only one third of patients with rheumatic fever.

### Treatment

There is no evidence that prolonged bed-rest shortens the course of acute rheumatic fever or reduces valvular damage. Early penicillin therapy may modify the course of the disease and a single intramuscular injection of benzathine penicillin in a dose of 1 200 000 units is recommended. Salicylates provide effective control of fever and the pain of arthritis in doses of 100 mg/kg/day. Prednisone in a dose of 2 mg/kg/day should be reserved for patients with severe carditis, cardiac failure and pericarditis. The dose must be reduced gradually over a period of weeks.

# *Chronic rheumatic heart disease*

## Mitral stenosis

It usually takes 20 years for significant stenosis to develop following the acute attack of rheumatic fever. Symptoms may appear in the twenties and become incapacitating within 10 years, and include dyspnoea, paroxysmal nocturnal dyspnoea with orthopnoea, fatigue, haemoptysis, systemic emboli, congestive cardiac failure, recurrent pulmonary infection, angina and pleuritic pain due to pulmonary infarction.

On examination 70 per cent of pregnant patients with rheumatic valve disease have the physical signs of mitral stenosis which include mitral facies, atrial fibrillation, a raised jugular venous pulse, a diastolic thrill at the apex together with a loud first sound, opening snap and a rumbling mid diastolic murmur best heard at the apex. The majority of patients with mild or moderate disease have uneventful pregnancies but the main complications, which are seen in those with severe rhuematic heart disease, include:

### Heart failure

This results from obstructed cardiac output rather than myocardial failure. Prompt treatment is essential and includes the administration of oxygen, a rapidly acting diuretic intravenously and slow digitalization. If these measures fail endotracheal intubation with assisted respiration should be considered. Surgery may be unavoidable and closed mitral valvotomy or mitral valve replacement have both been done in pregnancy. Indications for surgery include an attack of pulmonary oedema, haemoptysis and significant pulmonary hypertension. If surgery is considered during pregnancy the middle trimester appears to be the safest time for the fetus. During the first trimester the fetus is at risk from teratogenic hazards and abortion and in the third trimester there is an appreciable risk of precipitating premature labour or causing intra-uterine death.

### Disorders of cardiac rhythm

These are common in pregnancy and even occur in the absence of organic heart disease. Atrial tachyarrhythmias associated with rheumatic heart disease are important because they influence maternal morbidity and maternal and fetal mortality. Ventricular tachycardia is uncommon in pregnancy.

1. *Atrial fibrillation*. This only occurs at an advanced stage of rheumatic mitral valve disease in pregnancy. It usually develops after the fourth month of gestation when the blood volume is almost at its maximum and indicates significant myocardial damage. It is associated with a high incidence of heart failure and systemic embolism. Digitalis therapy controls atrial fibrillation but may make subsequent electroconversion to sinus rhythm difficult. The chances of sinus rhythm being maintained are dependent on the duration of the abnormal rhythm, left atrial size and the patient's age.

   Electroconversion is the method of choice in pregnancy and there is a 90 per cent chance of success; otherwise digoxin may be used to control the heart rate.

2. *Atrial flutter*. This is uncommon in pregnancy and is most suitably treated by electroconversion.

3. *Paroxysmal atrial tachycardia*. In the presence of organic heart disease atrial tachycardia can rapidly precipitate heart failure. If carotid massage and antidysrhythmic drugs are unsuccessful DC electrical cardioversion becomes necessary.

**Embolism**

Systemic embolism is ususally associated with mitral stenosis. The use of anticoagulants to prevent systemic embolism is controversial, but it does seem to reduce the number of embolic events.

# Other rheumatic valve diseases in pregnancy
## Mitral incompetence

Even in severe mitral regurgitation left ventricular failure is uncommon in pregnancy.

## Aortic incompetence

Pregnancy is well tolerated even in severe aortic incompetence, but pulmonary oedema due to left ventricular failure may develop.

## Aortic stenosis

This is compatible with normal cardiac function for a long time. Symptoms such as paroxysmal dyspnoea, effort angina and syncope tend to appear late in the course of the disease and are associated with a reduced life expectancy.

Pregnancy appears to be tolerated well by patients with rheumatic aortic stenosis.

## Prophylaxis of bacterial endocarditis

There is considerable controversy regarding the role of antibiotics in prevention of bacterial endocarditis. (Szekely and Snaith, 1974, Lowry and Steigbigel, 1978 and McDonald, 1979). The data from the *Confidential Maternal Mortality Reports* suggest that women with valve disease are at risk of developing endocarditis. Antibiotics should consequently be used to cover labour in women who are at risk. Five hundred mg ampicillin and 80 mg gentamicin intramuscularly every 8 hours has been recommended by de Swiet and Fidler, (1981). Patients who are penicillin-sensitive should receive an intravenous injection of 500 mg of vancomycin (Durack, 1975).

# Pregnancy in patients after valve replacement

The experience of cardiologists throughout the United Kingdom in the management of patients who become pregnant after valve replacement was recently reviewed (Oakley and Doherty, 1976). Thirty nine pregnancies in 34 women gave rise to 30 healthy babies. There were three spontaneous early abortions in women taking warfarin and one abortion occurred at 24 weeks in a patient who was not on anticoagulants. There were two late intra-uterine deaths, both in women receiving phenindione.

While many patients with aortic valve replacement for congenital or post-infective disease have nearly normal cardiac function most patients with rheumatic mitral or multivalvular disease still have considerable impairment of their cardiac function after surgery and many have atrial fibrillation. However, most patients including those with triple valve replacement, can cope easily with the demands of pregnancy.

The general care of these patients during pregnancy does not differ in principle from that of patients with valvular disease, but without valve replacement; although fetal mortality may be higher due to the use of oral anticoagulants. There is a real risk of systemic embolism if anticoagulants are withdrawn. This risk is less with modern prostheses and there appears to be no need for anticoagulation with tissue valve replacements.

Heparin may be given during the first trimester and then oral anticoagulants substituted until 2 to 3 weeks before term when heparin is reintroduced. (Hirsch *et al*, 1970). Oral anticoagulants are re-established after delivery. Their presence in breast milk is not a significant problem. However, all babies born to such mothers should receive vitamin $K_1$ at birth.

# Infective endocarditis

The clinical manifestations of infective endocarditis are variable and early diagnosis can be difficult. There are three main features – infection, embolism and cardiac involvement. Malaise, fever, sweating and rigors occur and the fever is often remittent. Clubbing of the fingers and toes develops within weeks. Petechiae in the skin, mucous membranes, conjunctivae and fundi are associated with prolonged illness. Splinter haemorrhages under the nails occur but as they are also seen in otherwise healthy people as the result of trauma, their diagnostic importance is lessened. Cutaneous embolic phenomena occur on the finger and toe pads (Osler's nodes) and similar lesions on the palms and soles are eponymously called Janeway's lesions. Major thromboembolic episodes are less frequent following the introduction of antibiotics. Septic embolism may lead to mycotic aneurysms of the intracranial vessels, abdominal aorta or coronary arteries. The development of a new murmur is of more significance in reaching a diagnosis than is a change in the character of an existing murmur.

When reported as a complication of pregnancy or the puerperium the pathogens most frequently involved are commensals of the genital tract – Gram-negative organisms and anaerobic streptococci.

## Investigation

The most important finding is a bacteraemia. Unfortunately, negative blood cultures may occur in a quarter of patients and treatment may have to be instituted without laboratory confirmation when the diagnosis seems likely on clinical grounds. Five or six blood cultures should be obtained in order to avoid the misleading interpretation of a questionable single contaminated culture. The skin should be prepared with 70 per cent alcohol and iodine and the area should be punctured without retouching. If penicillin has been administered penicillinase should be added to the culture medium together with the blood sample.

## Treatment

Successful prophylaxis will prevent the development of bacterial endocarditis. Once established, treatment should be rapid and with bactericidal agents given parenterally. Treatment must be prolonged

and should never be less than 2 weeks for penicillin-sensitive streptococci nor less than 4 weeks for enterococcal infections. Once the
appropriate therapy is instituted, daily blood cultures and frequent
monitoring of serum bactericidal activity is advisable. A serum
bactericidal activity at a 1-in-8 or greater dilution is acceptable.

# Congenital heart disease

Most patients with acyanotic congenital heart disease, even in a
surgically uncorrected state, tolerate the haemodynamic burden of
pregnancy satisfactorily and have uneventful pregnancies.

## Persistent ductus arteriosus

This malformation is a common one, symptoms occurring as the
pulmonary artery pressure rises. If it is normal, patients are
asymptomatic but have a loud continuous machinery murmur. The
main risks in pregnancy are the development of heart failure or
bacterial infection. If heart failure develops, closure of the duct is
feasible during pregnancy. If the duct becomes infected, early closure
is advisable but antibiotic treatment should be started at once.

In patients in whom closure of the duct has been carried out prior to
pregnancy, the course of the pregnancy will be uncomplicated but
antibiotics should be given prophylactically during labour.

## Atrial septal defect

This is one of the most frequent congenital forms of heart disease. In
uncomplicated atrial septal defect the left-to-right shunt results in an
additional load on the right ventricle and an increased pulmonary
blood flow. Uncorrected atrial septal defect seldom leads to heart
failure or atrial dysrhythmias before the third or fourth decades.
Infective endocarditis is a rare complication.

The great majority of patients tolerate pregnancy well. If heart
failure develops during pregnancy, closure of the defect is indicated
without delay. Pregnancies occurring subsequent to closure of the
defect have been, on the whole, uneventful.

## Ventricular septal defect

This common abnormality may be asymptomatic if the defect is not
too large and the pulmonary vascular resistance normal. However,
with a large defect and normal pulmonary vascular resistance,

cardiac failure may appear in the third or fourth decade. If there is a high pulmonary resistance, transient or permanent cyanosis may develop due to the reversal of the shunt. There is a significant risk of bacterial endocarditis developing in all groups of patients. Surgical correction of the defect during pregnancy is rarely required.

In the immediate postpartum period there is a potential risk of reversal of the shunt if severe arterial hypotension occurs. Prompt action is necessary to restore the blood pressure to normal.

# Right-to-left shunts

## Fallot's tetralogy

For almost a century, this term has been applied to the combination of ventricular septal defects, pulmonary stenosis, an overriding aorta and right ventricular hypertrophy. The severity of the pulmonary stenosis determines the symptoms and the degree of cyanosis. In the past, few women reached child-bearing age, dying from heart failure, respiratory infection, bacterial endocarditis or cerebral complications. Antibiotic therapy and palliative or even corrective surgery have improved the prognosis. However, pregnancy presents a considerable risk to the mother and fetus. Unfavourable features include repeated syncopal attacks, a haematocrit over 60 per cent peripheral arterial oxygen saturation under 80 per cent and a right ventricular pressure exceeding 120 mmHg. Because of the serious risk of hypoxia to the fetus the mother must exert herself as little as possible during the first and third trimesters. The immediate postpartum period is most hazardous and fatal syncopal attacks have been reported at this time because of an abrupt increase in right-to-left shunt.

## Eisenmenger's disease

The original description was of a large ventricular septal defect with cyanosis which was erroneously attributed to streaming of blood from the right ventricle into an overriding aorta. It is now realized that the cyanosis is due to a right-to-left shunt at atrial, ventricular or aorto-pulmonary level, produced by pulmonary hypertension. A wide variety of malformations may therefore be associated with the syndrome. Cyanosis and evidence of pulmonary hypertension are invariably present. The right ventricle is palpable along the sternal edge, and the pulmonary component of the second sound may be felt in the second left interspace.

This congenital defect can be associated with a particularly high maternal mortality. Most patients die in the puerperium, due to a slowly falling arterial oxygen saturation associated with a decrease in cardiac output. Although termination is advisable, if the woman wishes to continue with the pregnancy prophylactic anticoagulation should be considered (De Swiet and Fidler, 1981). Labour is probably best managed with epidural anaesthesia and if the patient deteriorates she may need oxygen and $\alpha$ sympathomimetic amines such as noradrenaline.

# Primary valvular and vascular abnormalities

## Coarctation of the aorta

In this condition a localized or diffuse narrowing of the aorta varying from complete obstruction to trivial narrowing of the lumen occurs. Systolic and diastolic hypertension of the upper limbs is present. When palpable the femoral pulses are delayed.

Most women have successful pregnancies, although there is some risk of rupture of the aorta or dissection. Delivery should be by the vaginal route. Pregnancies subsequent to successful resection of the coarctation are usually uneventful.

## Primary pulmonary hypertension

Primary pulmonary hypertension is associated with a high total pulmonary vascular resistance and a normal pulmonary wedge pressure so that the obstruction to blood flow is proximal to the pulmonary capillary bed. There is a low and probably fixed cardiac output. Progression of the disease is especially rapid in younger patients.

The symptoms of shortness of breath, chest pain and syncope are aggravated by pregnancy, which contributes a serious risk to maternal life. A maternal mortality as high as 53 per cent has been reported (Morgan Jones and Howitt, 1965). Labour and the puerperium are the most critical periods and patients usually die from sudden circulatory collapse.

## Hypertrophic obstructive cardiomyopathy

Symptoms usually develop in the third and fourth decade and exertional dyspnoea, angina, fatigue and dizziness predominate. Syncope and congestive cardiac failure carry a poor prognosis. Physical examination reveals brisk, jerky pulses and left ventricular hypertrophy. A mid systolic ejection murmur is best heard along the left sternal edge.

The outcome of 54 pregnancies in 23 patients with hypertrophic cardiomyopathy was analyzed by Oakley *et al* (1979). No mother or infant died in the perinatal period. Six patients developed dyspnoea which required treatment with diuretics. β-blockers were given in 18 pregnancies and three of the infants in this group were small-for-dates and in two, fetal bradycardia occurred. These results confirmed the safety of pregnancy in patients with hypertrophic cardiomyopathy. Delivery should be by the vaginal route and epidural anaesthesia avoided because of the risk of hypotension. Antibiotic prophylaxis against endocarditis is essential. The decision to administer a β-blocker must be made in individual cases; they should be given for relief of angina but otherwise avoided.

# *Myocardial and pericardial disorders*

## Cardiomyopathy of pregnancy

This condition may either be a specific disease of pregnancy or simply represent the effects of untreated hypertension or malnutrition. The majority of patients develop symptoms during the 3 months following delivery and are usually breast feeding their children. Women are often over 30 years of age and of tropical or negro origin. The main features are of sudden development of dyspnoea, chest pain, haemoptysis, cardiomegaly, congestive cardiac failure, arrhythmias and emboli, particularly to the lungs. Pulmonary embolism is an important cause of death, which occurs in up to 60 per cent of patients.

### Investigation

The electrocardiogram shows non-specific changes with low voltage QRS complexes and flat or inverted T waves over the surface of the left ventricle and there may be atrioventricular or intraventricular conduction defects. These changes regress slowly and can persist for 6 months. Chest radiology shows a gross cardiomegaly involving all chambers of the heart.

### Treatment

In patients with heart failure, treatment consists of bed-rest, digoxin, diuretics and sodium restriction. In view of the high incidence of thromboembolism anticoagulant therapy should be considered.

The long term prognosis is variable. Of those who survive the initial episode of heart failure, most recover fully but some show progressive disability and recurrence may occur after subsequent pregnancies.

# Myocardial infarction and pregnancy

Myocardial infarction is rare in women of child-bearing age. Ginz (1970) estimated that the incidence of acute cardiac infarction in pregnancies was about 1 in 10 000 deliveries. There was an overall mortality of 28 per cent, the highest mortality occurring in the puerperium.

## Investigation

Complaints of high abdominal discomfort or pain are commonly associated with hiatus hernia in pregnancy which may confuse the diagnosis. Lactic dehydrogenase levels are often elevated in pregnancy. ST segment changes and T wave flattening may occur because of positional changes in a normal pregnancy. The diagnosis of cardiac infarction is consequently difficult.

## Treatment

When myocardial infarction occurs in pregnancy, treatment is the same as for the non-pregnant patient with management on a coronary care unit. The earlier the infarct occurs during the pregnancy, the better the prognosis.

## Further reading

Batson, G.A. (1974). Cyanotic congenital heart disease and pregnancy. *Journal of Obstetrics and Gynaecology of the British Commonwealth* **81**, 549.

Ginz, B. (1970). Myocardial infarction in pregnancy. *Journal of Obstetrics and Gynaecology of the British Commonwealth* **77**, 610.

Morgan Jones, A. and Howitt, G. (1965). Eisenmenger syndrome in pregnancy. *British Medical Journal* **1**, 1627.

Oakley, D.G., McGarry, K., Limb, D.G. and Oakley, C.M. (1979). Management of pregnancy in patients with hypertrophic cardiomyopathy. *British Medical Journal* **1**, 1749.

## References

De Swiet, M. and Fidler, J. (1981). Heart disease in pregnancy: some controversies. *Journal of the Royal College of Physicians of London* **15**, 183.

Hirsh, J., Cade, J.F. and O'Sullivan, E.F. (1970). Clinical

experience with anticoagulant therapy during pregnancy. *British Medical Journal* **1**, 270.

Oakley, C.M. and Doherty, P. (1976). Pregnancy in patients after valve replacement. *British Heart Journal* **38**, 1140.

Szekely, P. and Snaith, L. (1974). *Heart Disease and Pregnancy*. Churchill and Livingston, Edinburgh.

# 4

# Diseases of the respiratory system

## Physiological changes

Minute ventilation is increased by about 40 per cent in pregnancy due to an increase in tidal volume, rather than an increase in respiratory rate. The increase in ventilation in excess of oxygen consumption and carbon dioxide production may produce a mild respiratory alkalosis. There is usually a compensatory metabolic acidosis. This ventilatory increase which is inappropriate to demand, may explain why some normal women feel breathless in pregnancy. Although pregnancy increases oxygen requirements by 25 per cent, respiratory failure is rare even in those women with diseased lungs, indicating that ventilatory reserve is considerable.

Dyspnoea is probably the most common complaint of the respiratory tract seen during the first 28 weeks of gestation. Up to 70 per cent of women complain of mild breathlessness which does not seem to affect their day to day activities.

**Table 4.1** Changes in lung function during pregnancy

| Anatomical changes | | | |
|---|---|---|---|
| | 1. | Average circumference of thoracic cage increased by 5 to 7 cm | |
| | 2. | Antero-posterior and transverse diameters increased | |
| | 3. | Substernal angle increased from 68° to 104° | |
| | 4. | Reduction in vertical diameter of the thorax by 4 cm | |

| Radiological changes | | |
|---|---|---|
| | 1. | Chest X-rays show an increase in lung markings which may simulate congestive heart failure |

*Physiological changes*

| | First trimester | Second trimester | Third trimester |
|---|---|---|---|
| Minute ventilation | Early increase | Increased | Increased by 150 % |
| Tidal volume | Increased | Increased | Increased by 125–140 % |
| Forced expiratory volume | ← | Increased | → |
| Respiratory rate | ← | Little change | → |
| Peak flow rate | ← | Little change | → |
| Functional residual capacity | ← | Decreased | → |
| Inspiratory reserve | ← | Decreased | → |

| Acid–base chemistry | | |
|---|---|---|
| | 1. | Plasma carbon dioxide reduced (p $CO_2$ = 30–32 mmHg) |

# Bronchial asthma

Asthma is characterized by paroxysms of expiratory dyspnoea and wheezing with overinflation of the lungs. Attacks are of variable duration and between attacks pulmonary function is normal so that patients are relatively symptom free. Episodes of asthma may last from minutes to several hours, but occasionally they may last days and some patients have problems with airway obstruction almost every day. The essential diagnostic feature is that the condition is reversible.

The narrowed bronchi and increased amounts of tenacious sputum make wheezing a prominent physical sign in both inspiration and expiration. The sputum is usually mucoid and white and contains no blood or pus, but may contain eosinophils and mucus casts of the smaller bronchi (Curschmann's spirals).

Prolongation of an asthmatic attack which does not respond to conventional therapy is classified as status asthmaticus. The patient becomes exhausted with the effort of breathing. If this is unrelieved respiratory acidosis supervenes and possibly death. Asthmatic episodes are sometimes complicated by atelectasis due to mucoid plugging of bronchi with subsequent absorption of gases. Spontaneous pneumothorax may also occur.

Pregnancy has no consistent effect on asthma. In a study of American negroes, babies tended to be premature and small with a perinatal mortality of 6 per cent. This finding has not been confirmed in Britain where the risk to the fetus is small.

## Investigations

Measurements of pulmonary function demonstrate decreased air flow, increased airway resistance and hyperinflation which are almost completely reversible between attacks and are improved by bronchodilators. No single test is diagnostic of asthma.

## Treatment

The pregnant patient with asthma should avoid known allergens as far as is possible. Attempts should be made to relieve anxiety. Infective episodes demand sputum culture and appropriate antibiotic therapy. Pregnancy does not provide particular problems in the normal medical management of the asthmatic patient.

Although $\beta$ stimulant bronchodilators such as salbutamol may theoretically prolong pregnancy because they inhibit uterine contraction and have been used to stop premature labour, they do not have a significant effect on normal labour. Patients with a true allergic precipitant for their asthma respond to disodium cromoglycate which inhibits mast cell degranulation. It has no demonstrated teratogenic effect. Inhaled steroids such as beclomethasone are also well tolerated.

Status asthmaticus in non-pregnant patients is particularly lethal and this is no different during pregnancy. Patients in status asthmaticus should be managed by physicians who would normally employ nebulized salbutamol, high dose steroids, adequate fluid replacement and where necessary artificial ventilation. In pregnancy a $PCO_2$ of greater than 35 mmHg or a pH of less than 7.35 should alert the physician to the possible need for ventilation. If the arterial $PO_2$ drops below 60 mmHg the fetus is at risk and delivery by Caesarian section should be considered, especially if the pregnancy is at term.

### Management of labour

Patients who have received steroids during the previous year require steroid cover. The following regime has been suggested by de Swiet (1977).

1. 100 mg hydrocortisone i.m. 6 hourly during labour.
2. Rapid reduction of steroids during the 48 hours after delivery.
3. Delivery should be vaginal provided there are no obstetrical contraindications.

# Bronchitis and emphysema

Chronic bronchitis is characterized by excessive mucus production in the bronchial tree resulting in regular frequent expectoration of sputum for at least 3 months of the year for 2 consecutive years. There is considerable hypertrophy of the mucus secreting glands which results in a disturbance of ventilation with increased airways resistance and eventually hypercapnia and hypoxia.

In emphysema the patient usually has a history of shortness of breath but only a small amount of mucus is produced. The chest is hyperresonant to percussion with reduced breath sounds and an increase in total lung capacity.

The occurrence of pregnancy in patients with chronic bronchitis has increased in recent years due to increased smoking habits of women. Chronic obstructive airways disease occurs only after many years of smoking and chronic bronchitis is still an unusual feature of pregnancy. Apart from its effects on maternal lung function, smoking has serious effects on the fetus.

### Investigations

The most reliable sign of airway obstruction is a prolongation of the time to perform a forced expiration – the forced expiratory time

**Table 4.2** Possible effects of smoking on pregnancy and the fetus

| | |
|---|---|
| 1. *Pregnancy* | |
| | Spontaneous abortion |
| | Antepartum haemorrhage |
| 2. *Fetus* | |
| | Intra-uterine growth retardation and fetal death |
| | Prematurity |

There is some evidence that if a woman stops smoking by her fourth gestational month the risk of delivering a child whose birth-weight is low is no greater than in the non-smoker.

(FET). The time taken to expire forcibly from a position of complete inspiration usually takes 3 seconds; if it exceeds 6 seconds there is significant airway obstruction.

## Treatment

Naturally the mother should be encouraged to stop smoking. Patients with uncomplicated bronchitis require no special management. However, in severe cases, inhalational anaesthesia should, if possible, be avoided because of the risk of subsequent pulmonary collapse and infection. If bronchitis is complicated by severe pulmonary hypertension then maternal mortality is increased and termination may be necessary.

## Sarcoidosis

Fever, weight loss and fatigue are often non-specific presenting symptoms. Erythema nodosum is also associated with the presentation of sarcoidosis. Pulmonary involvement is the most common manifestation and is an indication for treatment. Varying degrees of dyspnoea and cough are present, although sputum is scanty. Physical findings are variable and non-specific. Respiratory excursion may be limited; crackles are heard at the lung bases. In some patients sarcoidosis is a chronic progressive disease and pulmonary insufficiency and cor pulmonale occur as late features.

Skin lesions occur in about a third of patients and affect the nose, eyes and mouth and vary from extensive erythema and raised lesions to small non-descript plaques and papules. These are often found at old scar sites.

In about three-quarters of cases the liver is involved, but only one third of cases have hepatomegaly and mild jaundice. This may rarely be associated with splenomegaly.

An acute granulomatous uveitis can be the initial manifestation of sarcoidosis. Ocular disease may progress to severe visual impairment and blindness with corneal opacities and secondary glaucoma. Lacrimal enlargement, conjunctival infiltration and keratoconjunctivitis sicca of the type seen in Sjogren's syndrome are common.

The disease has no ill effect on pregnancy and is not transmitted to the fetus. Patients who are symptom free require no treatment during pregnancy and serial chest X-rays usually show no advance of the disease. However, the puerperium may be a critical period in which therapy is necessary.

## Investigations

### Biochemical abnormalities

Hypergammaglobulinaemia and reduction of serum albumin are common. Hypercalcaemia and hypercalciuria may occur, but are unusual.

### Radiology

About 90 per cent of patients eventually show intrathoracic disease on chest X-ray. Bilateral hilar lymphadenopathy is a common feature and may be associated with diffuse parenchymal changes or pulmonary fibrosis.

### Kveim reaction

In 50–80 per cent of patients with sarcoidosis the intracutaneous injection of a heat-sterilized suspension of human sarcoid tissue from the spleen or lymph nodes produces a papulonodular lesion with epithelioid tubercles. The nodule must be biopsied in 4 to 6 weeks for routine histology. A false positive result occurs in about 1 per cent of normal people.

## Treatment

In about 90 per cent of patients presenting with erythema nodosum and hilar lymphadenopathy the lesions resolve spontaneously within two years. The resolution rate is slightly less in those who present with asymptomatic hilar lymphadenopathy or respiratory symptoms, about 20 per cent of whom develop pulmonary infiltrates with or without intrathoracic manifestations of sarcoidosis. Asymptomatic hilar adenopathy should not be treated. If there are symptoms or evidence of impaired lung function within 6 to 12 months of onset, steroid therapy in high doses for prolonged periods is indicated. Steroids prevent new granulomata forming and may accelerate clearing. In practise they are used to relieve symptoms, clear dense infiltrates and improve lung function. They probably do not effect established fibrosis which is associated with a mortality of about 70 per cent.

Exacerbations of the disease are rare in pregnancy. However, the puerperium may be a critical period in which steroids are necessary. This is particularly true if they have been used in treatment of the condition during the preceding two years. The obstetric management of pregnancy, labour and delivery does not differ from that of a normal patient.

# Cystic fibrosis

This autosomal recessively inherited condition results in chronic pulmonary disease, intestinal malabsorption due to pancreatic insufficiency and elevated concentrations of sodium and chloride in the sweat. Of these, it is usually pulmonary disease that determines the eventual outcome. The least severely affected patient has no cough and examination of the chest may be normal. Most patients, however, develop a persistent cough in childhood, associated with repeated infections, haemoptysis, pneumothorax and right-sided cardiac failure. More patients with cystic fibrosis now survive into their twenties and some of them have become pregnant.

Faecal impaction, intussusception and recurrent rectal prolapse may also be a problem and about 80 per cent of patients have pancreatic insufficiency which results in malabsorption with frequent loose stools. Diabetes and excessive loss of sodium and chloride in the sweat has led to metabolic problems.

## Investigation

### Radiology

Early in the disease, chest X-rays can be normal. The earliest radiological changes are accentuation of the bronchovascular markings particularly in the upper lobes. There may be lobular or lobar atelectases with or without pneumonitis. Emphysema can occur and areas of pneumonia or cavitated lesions are common.

In those patients with pancreatic insufficiency bone age may be retarded.

### Sodium and chloride in the sweat

The concentrations of both sodium and chloride in the sweat are over 70 mmol/litre in the patient with cystic fibrosis. These values are less reliable in adults; many normal people have values well above the diagnostic range.

## Treatment

Patients with cystic fibrosis are encouraged to lead as normal a life as possible and this includes pregnancy. The well-being of the patient with cystic fibrosis depends upon her day to day management at home which includes: active therapy of pulmonary complications, proper attention to good nutrition and salt replacement especially in hot weather.

### Respiratory complications

Physiotherapy is used to relieve bronchial obstruction due to accumulated secretions. It is needed on a daily basis even in patients with minimal disease. The patient places herself on a firm board that can be inclined to different angles for drainage of the middle lobe, lingula and basal sections of both lower lobes. The efficiency of this method may be improved by rendering the mucus less sticky by use of mucolytic drugs such as N-acetyl cysteine or aerosols.

During acute exacerbations of the disease intensive antibiotic therapy is mandatory to halt further deterioration. In pregnancy infection should be diagnosed early and the appropriate antibiotics chosen after sputum cultures.

### Nutritional support

This should include vitamins, pancreatic supplements and, if necessary, iron replacement. Diets should be high in both medium chain triglycerides and protein.

During pregnancy, maternal energy expenditure should be reduced by the use of bronchodilators and bed-rest. Adequate amounts of exogenous pancreatic exzymes should be provided as pancreatic enzyme supplements and the mother's nutrition may be monitored by serial measurements of serum albumin. The pregnancy should be continued as long as the mother's condition remains stable or as long as the vital capacity is maintained. Termination has been recommended when the vital capacity falls to 50 per cent of the normal value. Provided that the pelvis is adequate there is no contraindication to vaginal delivery. The risks of inhalational anaesthesia are many and epidural anaesthesia is the method of choice for operative procedures.

# Tuberculosis

In the past tuberculosis had a sinister reputation in pregnancy – patients often deteriorated in the puerperium. When it was recognized early in the pregnancy therapeutic abortion was often undertaken. Modern chemotherapy has significantly altered the outlook and relapses are no more frequent in patients who are pregnant than those who are not. Today, the disease is unusual in British-born women but is much more frequent in Asian women entering this country as immigrants. The incidence is particularly high in Pakistani women and less so in Indians. There appears to be no difference in the frequency of disease in West Indian and British-born women.

In most instances, the onset of chronic pulmonary tuberculosis is insidious and the patient may be entirely asymptomatic, the disease only being discovered on a routine chest X-ray. Fever, in the late afternoon or evening is common, with profuse sweating during sleep ('night sweats'). Significant weight loss occurs, usually in the later stages of the disease. Cough, sometimes associated with odourless sputum, which may be green or yellow in colour, is common. Haemoptysis sometimes supervenes. Physical examination may be unremarkable, hence the importance of chest radiology.

The disease has little effect on pregnancy. Spontaneous abortion is more frequent although premature labour does occur occasionally in patients with abdominal and active disease. However, women do appear to have an increased frequency of recurrence during the puerperium. This may reflect the disturbed nights, increased work and anxiety that follow the birth of a baby.

Experience with extrapulmonary tuberculosis in pregnancy is limited and early diagnosis is likely to be delayed.

## Investigations

### Radiology

The disease must be recognized early in pregnancy, as rapid deterioration may occur if appropriate treatment is not instituted. A full scale chest X-ray is needed, regardless of gestation, and adequate shielding of the abdomen should be provided. Miniature X-rays should not be used because of the high dose of radiation involved.

Some patients will show 'minimal lesions' on their chest X-rays (discrete, round opacities, less than a centimetre in diameter and usually situated in the upper zone). In about 20 per cent of cases, tubercle bacilli can be grown from laryngeal swabs or gastric contents. Because of this, chemotherapy should be given whilst awaiting the result of sputum culture and serial chest X-rays.

### Cultures

The only absolute proof of active tuberculosis is the culture of the organism. However, this is a prolonged process and a useful preliminary examination is to make a smear of the material and stain for acid-fast bacilli (Ziehl-Neelsen stain). The smear is insensitive but it has the virtue of quickly identifying a highly infectious patient who is excreting large numbers of organisms.

## Tuberculin skin tests

Tuberculin tests are less helpful in diagnosis than in non-pregnant patients. In some women with active disease the positive tuberculin test becomes negative as pregnancy advances ('anergic period').

# Treatment

The successful treatment of tuberculosis depends on an adequate course of therapy. Initially, three 'first line' antituberculous agents are given to prevent the emergence of a drug resistant strain of *Mycobacterium tuberculosis*. Treatment is modified once the sensitivities are known. Usually, two 'first line' drugs are used. Regular and prolonged chemotherapy is essential for the cure of this disease and patient cooperation is essential. For this reason, the treatment programme must be explained carefully to the pregnant woman and she must be reassured that her baby will not develop tuberculosis. Congenital tuberculosis is exceptionally rare.

## Chemotherapy during pregnancy

Initially, the treatment of tuberculosis should be: isoniazid (300 mg daily) and either PAS (16 g daily) or ethambutol (15 mg/kg daily). When sensitivities are known the appropriate drug should be selected (see Table 4.3). Once the first trimester is passed rifampicin and INAH may be used. Treatment should be continued for 9 months. Other regimes may involve treatment for as long as 1 or 2 years.

**Table 4.3** Drugs used to treat tuberculosis

| Drug | Dose | Maternal effects | Fetal effects |
|------|------|------------------|---------------|
| PAS | Oral 12 g daily | Bulky, poorly effective with gastro-intestinal side-effects | None reported but crosses placenta |
| Isoniazid | Oral, up to 300 mg daily | In high doses, peripheral neuritis which may be treated with 10–20 mg pyridoxine daily. | None reported but crosses placenta |
| Ethambutol | Oral 15 mg/kg daily | It may cause retrobulbar neuritis, red/green blindness and peripheral neuritis | No evidence that it is teratogenic |
| Rifampicin | Oral 450–600 mg daily | It may cause gastro-intestinal symptoms including jaundice and drug induced hepatitis | *Teratogenic in animals. Avoid in first trimester* |

Steroids may be required if the patient is acutely ill on presentation. They may also be required to suppress severe drug allergic reactions.

There is a significant risk that tuberculosis may be reactivated by pregnancy and patients who have received treatment during the previous 3 years should receive prophylactic therapy of INAH and rifampicin for the last 3 months of the pregnancy and the first 3 months of the puerperium.

## Chemotherapy during labour

This is not usually a problem unless the expectant mother is acutely ill. The patient usually has adequate ventilatory reserve; although forceps delivery is often prolonged due to reduced maternal effort. Patients are usually fit for inhalational anaesthesia if required, but the anaesthetic machine will need careful sterilization afterwards.

## Chemotherapy during the puerperium

Early in the pregnancy, the expectant mother with tuberculosis, should be warned of the precautions that are taken in the puerperium. She cannot feed or handle the baby, until her sputum has been sterilized and the baby vaccinated. Women with quiescent disease of less than 2 years duration should not feed their babies unless they are receiving prophylactic chemotherapy. The infants of all women who have active or inactive tuberculosis or who are returning to a home where there has been tuberculosis should receive BCG vaccination.

There is a significant risk of reactivation of recent tuberculosis during the puerperium and for this reason some authors believe that lactation should be suppressed, and *a chest X-ray performed a month after delivery*.

## The infant and BCG

The infant should receive BCG vaccination if the mother has been treated for tuberculosis or if there has been a case at the child's new home. If the organism was not resistant to isoniazid BCG should be used. The infant can stay with its mother, provided he or she receives 20 mg/kg isoniazid daily until the Mantoux reaction becomes positive. If the mother's organism is resistant to isoniazid, ordinary BCG should be given to the child and if she has open tuberculosis, the infant must be segregated from the mother until Mantoux conversion has occurred.

BCG vaccination is undertaken in the first week of life if the child weighs more than 2.3 kg. Smaller infants are at risk of local necrosis or abscess formation. The dose of vaccine used is 0.05 ml and is given intradermally at the junction of the upper and middle thirds of the deltoid muscle on the arm. Innoculation into the thigh is more often followed by abscess formation in the inguinal glands. Mantoux testing is carried out 6 weeks after innoculation, and, if negative, again 2 or 4 weeks later.

# Pulmonary complications of obstetric anaesthesia

Seven per cent of maternal deaths are due to complications of obstetric anaesthesia. The inhalation of solid gastric contents results in pulmonary collapse and infection while liquid gastric contents cause Mendelson's syndrome.

**Table 4.4**  Prevention of pulmonary complications of obstetric anaesthesia

---

*1. Postpartum pulmonary collapse*
  i.  Withhold solid food during labour
  ii.  Women who have had respiratory infections late in pregnancy should receive prophylactic antibiotics eg. 250 mg ampicillin orally qds
  iii.  Stop smoking
  iv.  Postoperative physiotherapy

*2. Mendelson's syndrome*
  i.  As above
  ii.  Regular antacid therapy every 3 hours
  iii.  Cimetidine given before induction of anaesthesia will raise the pH above the 'initial' value of 2.5 in the majority of patients. The agent may be given by oral, intramuscular or intravenous routes

---

## Postpartum pulmonary collapse

The first sign is usually the development of fever within 24 hours of the anaesthesia. If the area of collapse is large, the mediastinum will be displaced towards the affected side and an area of dullness to percussion may be identified. Crackles may be heard on auscultation.

## Investigations

A chest X-ray will show patchy areas of consolidation in the affected area. The diaphragm may be raised on the affected side. Lateral views should also be obtained as the consolidated area may be invisible behind the raised dome of the diaphragm.

## Treatment

Immediate physiotherapy is undertaken by doctor, nurse or physiotherapist. The patient is placed so that the affected lung is uppermost and the foot of the bed is raised by 2 feet. Forceful percussion is made over the collapsed area with the base of the palm. the patient is encouraged to make jerky expirations. If these techniques fail, emergency bronchoscopy to remove the solid material must be undertaken. Penicillin will be required and should be given parenterally.

# Mendelson's syndrome

There may be no signs of bronchial obstruction or pulmonary collapse. Over 2–6 hours the patient becomes dyspnoeic, wheezy and cyanosed. Tachycardia and hypertension are followed by pulmonary oedema.

## Investigation

Radiological examination shows small scattered opacities or fulminant pulmonary oedema.

## Treatment

Prevention is easier than treatment which consists of endotracheal intubation until the pulmonary oedema resolves. This may take a week. Intermittent positive pressure ventilation with 100 per cent oxygen may be required. Parenteral penicillin should be given prophylactically (1 mega unit 6 hourly). Two hundred mg of intravenous or intramuscular hydrocortisone should be given 6 hourly and intravenous frusemide (40 mg) may help in resolving the pulmonary oedema.

# Further reading

Barnes, C.G. (1974). *Medical Disorders in Obstetric Practice. Fourth Edition.* Blackwell Scientific Publications, Oxford.

Crawford, S. (1984). *Principles and Practice of Obstetric Anaesthesia.* Blackwell Scientific Publications, Oxford.

Leontic, E.A. (1977). Respiratory disease in pregnancy. *Medical Clinics of North America* **61**, 111.

de Swiet, M. (1977). Diseases of the respiratory system. *Clinics in Obstetrics and Gynaecology* **4**, 287.

de Swiet (1984). *Medical Disorders in Obstetric Practice.* Blackwell Scientific Publications, Oxford.

# 5

# Renal disease in pregnancy

As early as the third month of pregnancy, the mean effective renal plasma flow as measured by para-aminohippuric acid clearance (PAH) begins to increase and by the end of the fourth month is 30–40 per cent greater than in the non-pregnant patient. About the seventh month it begins to subside and probably at term is only slightly above the non-pregnant mean. Coincident with the increase in renal blood flow the glomerular filtration rate, as measured by inulin clearance also increases, and by the fourth month is over 50 per cent higher than the non-pregnant mean. Tubular reabsorption is unaffected by pregnancy.

**Table 5.1** Normal renal changes in pregnancy

| | |
|---|---|
| *Renal size* | The length increases by 1 cm |
| *Renal structure* | The calyces, pelvis and ureter dilate, increasing the chance of urinary stones asymptomatic bacteriuria and frank pyelonephritis<br>Dilatation persists until 12–16 weeks postpartum |
| *Renal function* | Glomerular filtration rate (GFR) is increased by an average of 50–100 % to 120 ml/min. This results in a fall in the levels of serum creatinine to 65 $\mu$mol/litre in the first trimester and 51 $\mu$mol/litre in the second. Hence, apparently normal non-pregnant levels may indicate disease in the pregnant woman. Levels of creatinine above 75 $\mu$mol/litre or of urea above 4.5 mmol/litre suggest the need for further evaluation<br>Excretion of glucose, most amino acids and several water soluble vitamins is increased<br>Urinary protein excretion is increased |

## Investigations

### Renal function tests

Urea and creatinine clearances do not measure absolute glomerular filtration rates (GFR) as urea is reabsorbed and creatinine is secreted by the tubules. However, they do provide an assessment of renal

**Table 5.2** Evaluation of renal function in pregnancy

| Function | Clinical test | Use in pregnancy |
|---|---|---|
| Glomerular filtration rate (GFR) | 1. Creatinine clearance<br>2. Urea clearance<br>3. Serum creatinine<br>4. Serum area nitrogen | 30–50 % above normal pregnant values means that there is significant renal disease |
| Distal tubular transport | 1. Concentration and dilution<br>2. Maximal and minimal specific gravities or osmolality | Normal values are probably similar to non-pregnant women. The sample should be obtained with the woman in the lateral recumbent position. |
| Acid-base metabolism | 1. Minimal urine pH after acid loading | Pregnant women often have urine with a pH above 5.5. Acid loading protocols *ARE SELDOM INDICATED IN PREGNANCY* |

function. Regular measures of creatinine clearance through pregnancy are important in patients with renal disease. Uric acid measurements are of particular use in pre-eclampsia. There is reduced clearance with a consequent rise in plasma urate and this precedes any change in creatinine or urea.

Urine should be examined for casts and protein, as in non-pregnant patients. They probably have the same significance, but excessive proteinuria may indicate pre-eclampsia provided pyelonephritis has been excluded.

**Renal biopsy**

Although the risks of biopsy during pregnancy are minimal, this procedure is usually delayed until the puerperium. One of the few indications for renal biopsy during pregnancy is nephrotic syndrome of unknown aetiology, occurring late in the second trimester or early in the third. At a later date, the fetus will probably be delivered successfully regardless of biopsy results.

## *Pregnancy in patients with pre-existing renal disease*

## Chronic glomerulonephritis

In the past, many patients with essential hypertension or chronic pyelonephritis have been diagnosed as suffering from chronic nephritis and without renal biopsy the distinction may be impossible. A past history of haematuria or oedema points towards nephritis, as does fetal death in the early weeks of previous pregnancies.

Glomerulonephritis is classified into the following groups:

### Minimal change glomerulonephritis

The glomeruli appear normal on light microscopy but electron microscopy reveals fusion of the foot processes of epithelial cells. It is relatively common and may present abruptly. Haematuria is not a feature. The disease responds to treatment with cyclophosphamide or steroids.

### Proliferative glomerulonephritis

The glomeruli show an increase in the numbers of one or more cellular elements. The increase in cellular numbers may be localized or diffuse. Epithelial cells are increased in the most severe form of glomerulonephritis where they lead to the formation of crescents. This rapidly progressive glomerulonephritis leads to renal failure within a few weeks or months. This type of glomerulonephritis is often associated with asymptomatic proteinuria.

### Membranous nephropathy

On light microscopy there is thickening of capillary basement membranes of the glomeruli. It is usually associated with heavy proteinuria over many years and is found in 15–20 per cent of adults with persistent proteinuria. If the proteinuria is sufficiently heavy, nephrosis supervenes. Hypertension is not a feature of this condition even when chronic renal failure develops.

### Membranoproliferative nephropathy

The glomeruli are moderately hypercellular, the capillary loops are thickened and later become lobulated. There is granular deposition of immunoglobulins and complement within the glomeruli. It usually presents in early adult life, especially in women and accounts for 25 per cent of cases with persistent proteinuria. Treatment is symptomatic. There is no evidence that steroids or immunosuppressants alter the course of the disease.

## Investigation

If proteinuria arises during pregnancy and bacteriuria and pre-eclampsia have been excluded, an attempt should be made to establish the diagnosis. An intravenous pyelogram should not be performed because of the risk to the fetus and without it a renal biopsy is difficult. It may be possible to perform the biopsy under ultrasonic guidance, but otherwise the investigation should be delayed until after delivery.

## Treatment

If the patient is receiving steroids they should be continued as necessary during the pregnancy. The patient usually develops oedema during the second half of pregnancy, but this may be controlled by adequate doses of diuretics e.g. 40–80 mg frusemide in the morning. Fluid intake is restricted and should equal the volume of urine excreted the previous day. Salty foods should be avoided so that only 60–80 mmol of sodium a day is ingested. Diet, however, should be high in protein. Pregnancy often exacerbates chronic glomerulonephritis, but rises in blood pressure, increases in oedema or other signs of eclampsia can be controlled and therapeutic abortion is seldom necessary. However, intra-uterine growth retardation is a common complication, often indicating early delivery.

# Polycystic disease

Adult polycystic disease tends to present between 20 and 40 years old. It is complicated by haemorrhage into renal cysts resulting in loin pain and haematuria, urinary tract infections, hypertension, subarachnoid haemorrhages and chronic renal failure. At this stage the kidneys are usually readily palpable.

## Investigation

The intravenous pyelogram is characteristic with bilateral renal enlargement with irregular outlines due to cysts. The calyces are compressed and elongated. However, ultrasound is obviously a preferable examination in pregnancy and the patient may even be diagnosed by abdominal palpation at the antenatal clinic.

## Treatment

Patients usually have an uncomplicated pregnancy, but as the condition has an autosomal dominant pattern of inheritance, genetic counselling is important.

# Chronic renal failure

The causes of chronic renal failure are legion. Symptoms do not usually develop until the urea is above 40 mmol/litre. The symptoms and signs are loosely termed the uraemic syndrome and are only seen to their full extent in patients with urea levels above 80 mmol/litre. The features of the disease include, pruritus, cutaneous pigmentation, sensory or motor neuropathies, osteomalacia and secondary hyperparathyroidism. Patients often have a normochromic (MCHC 32–36 per cent) and normocytic (MCVC 78–94 c$\mu$) anaemia.

There is little evidence that pregnancy has any effect upon the natural history of renal disease. Because of its insidious onset, chronic renal failure may first appear during pregnancy but escape diagnosis until hypertension is a problem in late pregnancy. Mild cases of renal failure present few problems during pregnancy apart from hypertension. In more severe cases, early transfer to a specialist unit with intensive care and dialysis facilities may be necessary.

## Investigation

Glomerulonephritis, malignant hypertension and chronic pyelo-nephritis are responsible for about 60 per cent of cases and polycystic renal disease and obstructive uropathies for about 15–20 per cent.

## Treatment

The major aim in therapy is to control symptoms and delay progressive renal damage. The measures usually adopted include; adequate fluid intake, control of hypertension and serum potassium. Anaemia may require treatment with larger doses of iron than is usual in pregnancy, or even a blood transfusion. Uraemic osteodystrophy may be aggravated by fetal requirements for calcium and can be recognized by an increase in the serum level of bony alkaline phosphatase. Serum calcium levels should be monitored, and if low, the patient may require 1 mg of alfacalcidol daily. Phosphate absorption can be controlled with oral aluminium hydroxide. Normally a diet of 40 g protein daily is recommended. In pregnancy, a 70 g intake is necessary because of fetal requirements.

Only if the renal failure is advanced will termination be necessary and even then intermittent haemodialysis in a specialist centre should be considered. Renal hypertension may, however, predispose to superimposed pre-eclampsia.

# Renal transplantation

Several hundred women who have had renal transplants have successfully completed their pregnancies. However, they tend to have problems with control of blood pressure, anaemia and recurrent urinary tract infections. Bone disease is common. Babies tend to be small-for-dates.

Transplant patients who wish to become pregnant should be in good general health for at least 2 years after transplantation and have no hypertension or proteinuria. They should show no evidence of graft rejection and, if on prednisone, the dose should be less than 15 mg/day. If azathioprine is being taken, the dose should be less than 200 mg daily. It is essential that the normal maintenance dosage of these drugs should be continued throughout pregnancy. The majority of patients with renal transplants have undergone vaginal delivery.

## *Renal disease arising during pregnancy*

## Acute glomerulonephritis

This syndrome is sudden in onset and characterized by haematuria and/or proteinuria possibly with a nephrotic syndrome. It is often associated with a haemolytic *Streptococcus* Group A infection 10 days previously.

### Investigation

There is a moderately raised blood urea and creatinine, the antistreptolysin O (ASO) titre is elevated and serum complement is initially low. The urinary sediment has many red blood cells, hyaline, granular and red cell casts.

### Treatment

Fluids must be restricted until diuresis begins. If oedema, pulmonary oedema or hypertension encephalopathy develop, diuretics will be needed. Steroids and cytotoxics are not required. Even though the syndrome usually disappears clinically in 1 week, abortion or delivery of a premature fetus may result. If renal disease is severe or persists for several weeks then termination is indicated.

## Nephrotic syndrome

This is a clinical state with a number of causes and it is characterized by increased glomerular membrane permeability resulting in heavy proteinuria (greater than 5 g/day) and the excretion of fat bodies. The urinary protein loss leads to hypoproteinaemic oedema. There is also a tendency to hyperlipidaemia.

**Table 5.3** Common causes of nephrotic syndrome

---

Diabetes
Amyloidosis
Systemic lupus erythematosus
Polyarteritis nodosa
Syphylis
Malaria
Renal vein thrombosis
Secondary to glomerulonephritis
Lipoid nephrosis

---

## Investigation

Because the treatments of the diverse causes of nephrotic syndrome are so different it is essential to establish a diagnosis.

## Treatment

There is no evidence that bed-rest ameliorates any features of nephrotic syndrome. If it is impossible to reverse the negative nitrogen balance, a diet containing 3 g of first class protein/kg of oedema free body weight must be provided. A rise in blood urea is acceptable provided it does not go above 40 mmol/litre. Sodium restriction may be necessary to control oedema but frusemide should be avoided as it may impair placental perfusion or increase the tendency to thrombotic episodes due to haemoconcentration. The majority of pregnancies reach term, although the infants tend to be small-for-dates, and there is some evidence that they have impaired neurological and mental development.

# Acute renal failure

A fall in urine output is usually the first sign of acute renal failure, with a volume of less than 400 ml/24 hours. It may be of three types:

### Prerenal failure

There are functional changes but no damage to the kidneys ie. urine output drops because of a failure in adequate renal perfusion. The causes include, severe haemorrhage, septicaemia, diabetes mellitus, hypertension with heart failure and prolonged vomiting. The circulating volume is usually reduced and a good response is often obtained with fluid replacement in haemorrhage, diabetes and vomiting.

**Intrinsic renal failure**

This implies renal damage, usually acute tubular necrosis. This may follow surgery, septic abortion, mismatched blood transfusion, acute glomerulonephritis or renal vein thrombosis. It can also be due to accidental haemorrhage associated with pregnancy. There is glomerular destruction which is seldom followed by return to normal function. At one time this was thought to be due to a 'uterorenal reflex', but it is probably caused by a combination of reduced perfusion and disseminated intravascular coagulation.

**Postrenal failure**

This is due to obstruction of the urinary tract and is often caused by urinary stones. Small stones are usually easily passed down the dilated tract of pregnancy but may lodge at the ureteric orifice. A plain abdominal film should be examined. An intravenous pyelogram may be of little help in pregnancy but cystoscopy and retrograde ureterograms may reveal the diagnosis.

## Intrinsic renal failure in pregnancy

The typical patient with acute renal failure in pregnancy has intrinsic renal disease and passes little urine for up to 14 days – acute tubular necrosis. This phase can last for 40 days. It is followed by a period of passage of increasingly large quantities of dilute urine – the diuretic phase. During this period, the urea falls to normal and subsequently urine returns to its normal concentration. However, acute cortical necrosis is not uncommon and this is followed by partial recovery.

Acute renal failure occurs in about 1 in every 2000–5000 pregnancies. Its frequency of distribution is bimodal with a peak in early pregnancy (12–18 weeks) and a second during the 35th–40th weeks. Cases occurring early in pregnancy are usually due to septic abortion and those later in pregnancy are usually associated with severe pre-eclampsia.

## Investigation

The patient has oliguria but the urine is isosmotic with plasma and has a value of 400–500 mOsm/litre. Urinary sodium is more than 70 mmol/litre and the urinary to plasma ratio for urea is less than 10. In the early stages plasma urea is of little help.

## Treatment

The underlying cause should be treated where it is known.

**Management of the initial stage**

The value of high dose diuretics (e.g. 500 mg frusemide) in reversing oliguria before acute tubular necrosis is established remains uncertain.

**Management of the established stage**

*A careful record of fluid intake and output must be maintained throughout the illness.*

*Hydration*
*The fluid requirement of an afebrile 70 kg patient is 500 ml daily plus the daily volume of urine and the volume lost from the gastrointestinal tract. Patients should be weighed daily and there should only be a slight increase in weight provided a correct fluid balance has been kept. The fluid does not need to be given intravenously.*

In severe pre-eclampsia or eclampsia with proteinuria, the patients are usually hypovolaemic and renal perfusion needs to be improved. These women can be grossly oedematous due to a compartmental shift in fluids. They will often respond well to a colloid infusion but the central venous pressure must be carefully monitored.

**Electrolyte control**
Sodium excess or deficiency is not usually a problem. Hyperkalaemia is a serious complication and if it exceeds 7 mmol/litre urgent treatment is essential to prevent cardiac arrest. It may be controlled by 10 ml of 10 per cent calcium gluconate intravenously, supported with oral or rectal calcium resonium (20–30 g, 4 to 8 hourly). Haemodialysis may be required at a specialist unit. In pregnancy, insulin and glucose should be used with caution.

*Nutrition*
The patient with renal failure loses weight and there is catabolism of body protein. She requires a high calorie (2500 calories or more) diet and also first class protein (20 g) daily.

When acute renal failure develops during pregnancy, intra-uterine death is a strong possibility, and early transfer to a specialist unit with intensive care and dialysis facilities should be arranged.

# Urinary tract infections

Urinary tract infection is one of the most common infectious complications of pregnancy. The investigative work of Kass has shown that significant bacteriuria can occur in the absence of symptoms or signs of urinary tract infection. He established quantitative bacteriology of mid-stream specimens as essential in the diagnosis of these infections and the presence of 100 000 or more colonies of a bacterial organism/millilitre of urine on two consecutive specimens indicated infection. This can occur in about 6 per cent prenatal patients and 40 per cent of these patients develop pyelonephritis.

Most women with asymptomatic bacteriuria are detected at the initial antenatal visit and relatively few women acquire bacteriuria later (1 per cent). Of these women between 20 and 40 per cent develop acute pyelonephritis during the pregnancy. If the bacteriuria is treated the incidence of pyelonephritis is significantly reduced by between 70 and 80 per cent. Pyelonephritis results in damage to tubular function and concentrating ability is consequently impaired. 10–15 per cent of pregnant women with bacteriuria develop chronic pyelonephritis some 10–12 years after delivery and 1 in 3000 pregnant women with bacteriuria ultimately develop chronic renal failure.

Bacteriuria is seen twice as frequently in pregnant women who are anaemic, although this has not been confirmed in all studies, and the anaemia may simply reflect chronic infection. The relationship between an increased incidence of hypertension in women with bacteriuria is also controversial. Pregnant women with bacteriuria who develop acute pyelonephritis have a significantly raised rate of prematurity. However, the relationship of prematurity and small-for-dates babies to asymptomatic bacteriuria is less clear cut. There is probably also an increased frequency of abortion and stillbirth and there is some evidence of a greater incidence of congenital malformations.

**Table 5.4** Features of bacteriuria in pregnancy

| | | |
|---|---|---|
| *Epidemiology* | 1. Increased frequency with age and parity — although some reports suggest the young primigravida is at greatest risk | |
| | 2. Increased frequency in indigent patients | |
| | 3. Increased frequency in patients with sickle cell trait | |
| | 4. Associated with anaemia | |
| *Bacteriology* | 1. *Escherichia coli* | 80 % |
| | 2. *Klebsiella — Enterobacter* | 10 % |
| | 3. *Proteus* | 5 % |
| | 4. *Pseudomonas* | |
| | 5. *Staphylococcus* | 15 % |
| | 6. Group D *Streptococcus* | |
| *Maternal complications* | 1. Acute pyelonephritis | |
| | 2. Anaemia | |
| | 3. Possibly an increased frequency of hypertensive disease of pregnancy | |
| | 4. Chronic pyelonephritis | |
| *Fetal complications* | 1. Prematurity | |
| | 2. Small-for-dates babies | |
| | 3. Increased frequency of abortions or stillbirths | |
| | 4. Increased incidence of dorsal mid-line fusion defects | |

## Investigation

Culture of mid-stream urine specimens will identify the infecting microorganism. It is possible to distinguish between renal and bladder infection with an immunofluorescent test for antibody-coated bacteria in the urinary sediment. In upper tract disease the bacteria are coated with antibody but this is not so with bladder infections.

Between 8 and 33 per cent of women with bacteriuria in pregnancy may subsequently be shown to have radiological changes consistent with chronic pyelonephritis and as many as 80 per cent have some renal tract abnormality.

## Treatment

Screening at the initial antenatal visit, appropriate treatment and eradication of bacteriuria will lead to the prevention of 70–80 per cent of all antenatal acute pyelonephritis. Treatment should be designed to maintain sterile urine throughout pregnancy with the shortest effective course of antibiotics. In the past, continuous antibiotic therapy has been used, but recent investigations suggest that short courses of 1–3 weeks duration are effective and even a single dose of 3 g of amoxycillin may be effective. Other drugs that have been used include:

1. *Short acting sulphonamides such as sulphafurazole.* These are best avoided in the last month of pregnancy because of the risk of unconjugated hyperbilirubinaemia and kernicterus. Co-trimoxazole should be avoided as it may cause congenital abnormalities in the first trimester, although this risk is a theoretical one.
2. *Nitrofurantoin.* This is of particular value in urinary tract rather than parenchymal infection. Resistance is unusual even after repeated or frequent use, but it does cause nausea and vomiting in as many as 20 per cent of patients.
3. *Nalidixic acid.* The possible role of this drug in producing hydrocephalus limits its use in pregnancy. This relationship is not clearly established and many pregnant women have received it without adverse effect.

Once acute pyelonephritis develops, hospital admission is indicated. The first choice antibiotic is amoxycillin given paranterally. If the patient does not respond rapidly, a broad spectrum cephalosporin should be substituted. Gentamicin has a limited role as it is ototoxic to the fetus. Once acute pyelonephritis has developed, appropriate suppressive therapy is indicated for the duration of the pregnancy.

# Renal tuberculosis

Renal tuberculosis usually presents as cystitis with frequency, dysuria haematuria and tenesmus.

## Investigation

The mid-stream urine reveals 'sterile' pyuria. Acid-fast bacilli may be demonstrated by Ziehl–Neelsen staining or by culture in guinea pigs, although this will take several weeks.

## Treatment

Since the advent of effective anti-tuberculous therapy termination is no longer indicated. Treatment is discussed in the chapter on respiratory disorders.

# Renal disease after pregnancy

## Acute postpartum renal failure

This most commonly follows postpartum haemorrhage. Its management is similar to that described earlier in this chapter. When dialysis is required it may be either peritoneal or haemodialysis. The choice depends upon the rate of rise of blood urea. If this exceeds 30 mmol/litre/day, peritoneal dialysis will not be sufficiently rapid.

### Technique of peritoneal dialysis

This may be undertaken in a side ward. The peritoneal space is entered with a disposable rigid catheter. If the patient experiences pain or there is ineffective return of dialysis fluid, the catheter is incorrectly placed and requires adjustment. With the catheter in place, sterile warm dialysis fluid is introduced in 1 to 2 litre aliquots. It is allowed to equilibrate ('dwell') and subsequently drained and discarded. Because of the long treatment time of 28–48 hours necessary with peritoneal dialysis, negative fluid balances of 10–15 litres may develop during this period and must be replaced orally or intravenously.

# Acute severe postpartum glomerulonephritis

This occurs during the puerperium and leads to severe oliguria. The patient may bleed from her mucous membranes and may die despite treatment. Those patients who survive usually have chronic renal failure with hypertension.

## Investigation

Renal biopsy shows severe proliferative glomerulonephritis with numerous crescents and the deposition of fibrin in the glomeruli.

## Treatment

The patient will require support with dialysis and may benefit from plasmaphoresis and possibly steroids or cyclophosphamide. However, the aetiology and effective treatment of this disease remain obscure.

# Further reading

Alvarez, R.R. (1978). Pre-eclampsia, eclampsia and renal diseases in pregnancy. *Clinical Obstetrics and Gynecology* **21**, 881.

Davison, J.M. and Lindheimer, M.D. (1978). Renal disease in pregnant women. *Clinical Obstetrics and Gynecology* **21**, 411.

McGeown, M.G. (1977). Renal disorders and renal failure. *Clinics in Obstetrics and Gynaecology* **4**, 319.

Polk, B.F. (1979). Urinary tract infection in pregnancy. *Clinical Obstetrics and Gynecology* **22**, 285.

Sweet, R.L. (1977). Bacteriuria and pyelonephritis during pregnancy. *Seminars in Perinatology* **1**, 25.

Wood, S.M. and Blainery, J.D. (1981). Hypertension and renal disease. *Clinics in Obstetrics and Gynaecology* **8**, 439.

# 6

# Endocrine diseases

## *Disorders of the pituitary gland*

## Pituitary tumours

Two groups of patients with pituitary tumours can be recognized in pregnancy.

1. Those with existing intrasellar or parasellar tumours who may have clinically evident endocrine disease. In the second half of pregnancy such women can develop visual restriction due to compression of the optic chiasma as the tumour expands. Vision usually recovers rapidly after delivery, but in severe cases it can only be preserved by the removal of the tumour during the pregnancy.
2. Microadenomas which cause selective gonadotrophin deficiency or hyperprolactinaemia. Pregnancy has been induced and the tumour enlarges. Any suggestion of an expanding lesion during pregnancy requires urgent investigation. Symptoms include headache and visual disturbance.

## Investigation

### Radiology

An enlarged pituitary fossa may be seen on a plain skull radiograph but patients with a microadenoma generally have a sella of normal size. Asymmetrical bulging of the sella floor in these patients is only revealed by thin cut tomography. A CT scan will detect a microadenoma which is larger than 6 mm and extends to the sella entrance or into the suprasellar of parasellar space. Cerebral angiography may be required to delineate the extension or exclude a carotid aneurysm.

### Ophthalmological investigation

Suprasellar extension of the tumour leads to compression of the optic nerve with resulting visual field defects and occasionally optic atrophy. Fifty per cent of cases have bitemporal hemianopia, though other defects such as central or nasal scotomas also occur, Papilloedema is only seen when the adenoma obstructs the foramen of Monro.

### Endocrine investigation

Basal hormone levels provide insufficient evidence to diagnose anterior pituitary failure. After obtaining a basal sample a combined dose of 100–200 micrograms thyrotrophin releasing hormone (TRH), 100 micrograms luteinizing hormone-releasing hormone (LH-RH) and 250 micrograms synthetic adrenocortico-trophic hormone (ACTH)(1–24 peptide) can be given and the second blood sample withdrawn thirty minutes after administration:

1. TRH stimulates thyroid stimulating hormone and prolactin secretion.
2. LH–RH stimulates luteinizing hormone (LH) and follicle stimulating hormone (FSH) secretion.
3. ACTH stimulates cortisol secretion and in 50 per cent of normal subjects growth hormone (GH) secretion.

If growth hormone secretion is to be measured accurately or if the patient has doubtful adrenal function an insulin hypoglycaemic test with 0.1–0.15 units/kg should be performed. GH releasing hormone is also undergoing clinical assessment.

## Acromegaly

Pregnancy in acromegaly is unusual. It should be allowed to continue as it does not affect the course of the disease and pregnancy is not adversely effected by the disease. Vision may deteriorate in later months, but usually recovers rapidly after delivery. Treatment is determined by the severity of the disease and the presence of complications. Infants born to acromegalic mothers tend to be above average weight but are otherwise healthy.

## Cushing's syndrome

*See* page 72

# Prolactinomas and pregnancy

The recognition and subsequent successful treatment of prolactin-producing tumours of the pituitary gland represents a comparatively new problem in obstetrics. Prior to the indentification of these tumours women would normally remain infertile or be rendered thus by treatment. Though experience of pregnancy in treated women is limited, it is possible to devise an effective protocol for surveillance and treatment of those at risk.

# Hyperprolactinaemic infertility

The principal cause of hyperprolactinaemia is excessive secretion from either a macro- or micro-adenoma of the pituitary gland, but there are others.

**Table 6.1** Causes of hyperprolactinaemia

| | |
|---|---|
| *Drugs* | Antiemetics (metoclopramide, domperidone) |
| | Antihistamines (meclozine, cimetidine) |
| | Antihypertensives (methyldopa, reserpine) |
| | Hormones (oestrogens, thyrotrophin-releasing factor) |
| | Narcotics (morphine) |
| | Psychotropics (chlorpromazine, imipramine, haloperidol, diazepam) |
| *Pituitary* | Prolactinoma |
| | Acromegaly |
| | Cushing's disease |
| | 'Empty sella' |
| *Hypothalamic* | Craniopharyngioma |
| | Pinealoma |
| *Others* | Primary hypothyroidism |
| | Chronic renal failure |
| | Idiopathic |

The most florid clinical presentation is of amenorrhoea, galactorrhoea and optic nerve compression. However, many women with the condition menstruate quite regularly and are only discovered during investigation of infertility. Clinical examination should exclude hypothyroidism or other causes of pituitary overactivity such as acromegaly of Cushing's disease. Visual field measurements may be reduced when large tumours compress the optic chiasma.

## Investigation

The diagnosis of hyperprolactinaemia is still controversial, but it is generally agreed that serum levels of greater than 850 mu/litre

(22 ng/ml) on three separate occasions establish the diagnosis. These levels are well below those usually encountered in the presence of micro-adenomas (mean levels of 5300 mu/litre (140 ng/ml), while macro-adenomas are associated with levels of 9800 mu/litre (260 ng/ml).

Once hyperprolactinaemia has been diagnosed and non-pituitary causes have been excluded, pituitary imaging is indicated. This can be achieved most accurately with high definition CT scanning. Lateral skull X-rays are still commonly used, sometimes in combination with sellar plane tomography. However, they are prone to misinterpretation as derangements of the sellar floor can be a normal variant.

## Treatment

Large tumours are usually treated medically. Dopaminergic drugs, in particular bromocriptine, are capable of producing a reduction in tumour size and inducing fertility in the great majority of patients. Neurosurgical and radiotherapeutic ablation of the pituitary gland have been historically important and may still be indicated in resistant and complicated cases.

### Management of bromocriptine-induced pregnancy

The majority of pregnancies achieved with bromocriptine progress smoothly, but there is a risk of tumour expansion or recurrence. This is particularly true for those with macro-adenomas where 2 per cent of cases develop such a complication. Prior knowledge of tumour size at diagnosis is consequently useful and patients should avoid conception until objective evidence of tumour regression has been recorded.

Throughout pregnancy, patients with macro-adenomas and probably those with micro-adenomas, should have monthly visual field measurements. Serum prolactin varies throughout pregnancy and cannot be used to monitor tumour recurrence. If recurrence occurs, bromocriptine must be restarted immediately and if visual fields continue to deteriorate emergency hypophyseal neurosurgery must be performed. The pregnancy may then be complicated by transient diabetes insipidus and spontaneous labour is less likely due to compromised oxytocin production.

Although bromocriptine may be safely used in pregnancy, the risk of tumour recurrence is not sufficient to warrant its use prophylactically. In the postpartum period it has been stated that drug treatment can be safely discontinued, that lactation is rapidly established and further tumour regression occurs. This may indeed be the case for the majority but appropriate surveillance throughout this period is strongly recommended.

# Hypopituitarism

This may be due to destruction of the pituitary by tumours or irradiation or from postpartum pituitary necrosis (Sheehan's syndrome). There is reduced fertility and in the untreated patient, pregnancy is rare. When pregnancy does occur, the first trimester is the critical period, after which it proceeds normally without pituitary activity. There is hypertrophy of any residual anterior pituitary tissue which may ameliorate the condition permanently or at least until delivery.

Hydrocortisone is required throughout pregnancy at a dose of about 30 mg daily. On the day prior to delivery and throughout labour 100–200 mg every 24 hours will be required and then rapidly reduced to the normal dose in the puerperium. Sufficient thyroxine is required to keep the serum thyroxine in the normal range.

# Diabetes insipidus

There are two types:

1. A deficiency of antidiuretic hormone – cranial diabetes insipidus.
2. Renal resistance to the action of antidiuretic hormone – nephrogenic diabetes insipidus.

# Cranial diabetes insipidus

Polyuria leads to hypertonic dehydration and polydipsia. Patients rely on thirst to maintain normal plasma osmolality. Menstruation and fertility are normal. Pregnancy may ameliorate or intensify symptoms or have no effect at all. Diabetes insipidus rarely develops during pregnancy but it may begin in the postpartum period.

## Investigation

Urine that remains hypotonic after fluid deprivation but is concentrated after exogenous vasopressin indicates cranial diabetes insipidus.

## Treatment

Patients with mild cranial diabetes insipidus (2–4 litres/24 hours) may require no specific therapy. Moderate or severe cranial diabetes insipidus usually responds to replacement therapy with desmopressin in a dose of 10–20 micrograms administered intranasally once or twice daily. Water intoxication may be avoided by adjusting the dose until the urine output is about 2 litres in 24 hours.

There is no known danger to the fetus from the disease and lactation is unaffected. Desmopressin is said to have no effect on uterine contractions.

# Nephrogenic diabetes insipidus

Any chronic renal disease may result in nephrogenic diabetes insipidus, although correction of electrolyte disturbances may restore sensitivity to antidiuretic hormone. There is also a sex-linked form of the disease which is associated with other renal tubular defects. Patients with this form of diabetes insipidus develop hypertonic dehydration and rely on their thirst mechanism to maintain plasma tonicity.

## Investigation

Hypotonic urine after exogenous antidiuretic hormone strongly suggests a diagnosis of nephrogenic diabetes insipidus. Plasma antidiuretic hormone levels are high but appropriate for the plasma osmolality whereas urine osmolality is inappropriately low.

## Treatment

Thiazide diuretics may be helpful. In the acquired form the underlying abnormality should be corrected as polyuria may be reversible. There appears to be no adverse effect on the fetus or management of the pregnancy.

# *Thyroid disorders*

Hypothyroidism may affect 9 in 1000 pregnancies and hyperthyroidism occurs in 2 in 1000 pregnant women. The recognition of these patients is important for the welfare of both mother and fetus. Important changes occur in the physiology of the thyroid gland during pregnancy and care must be taken in the interpretation of laboratory data.

## Thyroid physiology during pregnancy

During pregnancy, alterations occur in thyroid gland physiology and thyroid hormone transport. The renal threshold for iodine drops during pregnancy and consequently increased quantities of iodine are lost in the urine. This is particularly important when the dietary intake of iodine is low and a pregnancy goitre may result. The role of chorionic thyrotrophin and molar thyrotrophin in the production of pregnancy goitres is uncertain, but may explain why the thyroid-stimulating activity of the plasma is greater in pregnant than non-pregnant women. By the end of the first trimester the increased secretion of placental lactogen induces the liver to synthesize twice the normal amount of thyroxine binding globulin (TBG). The number of binding sites for $T_3$ and $T_4$ are increased and the total quantity of $T_3$ and $T_4$ is consequently in the 'thyrotoxic' range for non-pregnant women. A test for thyroid hormone binding such as $T_3$ resin uptake, detects the large number of vacant binding sites and gives a value in the 'hypothyroid' range. The free thyroxine index is derived from the total $T_4$ and $T_3$ resin uptake. It should be normal in pregnancy although there is a tendency for high values to be obtained.

Mother and fetus are fairly separate units as far as thyroid function is concerned. TSH does not cross the placental barrier and thyroid hormones pass across in very small quantities. However, antithyroid drugs such as carbimazole and propylthiouracil pass easily across the placenta, as do iodides and thyroid stimulating immunoglobulins.

## Diagnosis of thyroid disease in pregnancy

Normal pregnancy may mimic thyrotoxicosis because of the presence of goitre, heat intolerance, increased sweating, increased appetite, fatigue, tachycardia, palpitations, tremor and emotional lability. Hyperthyroidism may be evident because of weight loss or failure to gain weight normally, eye signs or pretibial myxoedema. By contrast, the weight gain of normal pregnancy may mask that due to hypothyroidism.

The following points must be borne in mind when interpreting biochemical investigations:

1. Serum TBG, $T_4$ and $T_3$ concentrations are highly variable with wide confidence limits.
2. Indirect measures such as free thyroxine index are often in the hyperthyroid range.
3. Although free thyroid hormone concentrations are not altered in pregnancy, direct assays of thyroxine may be inaccurate in the presence of an increased TBG concentration.

**Table 6.2** Thyroid tests in pregnancy (Modifed from Montgomery and Harley, 1977)

|  | *Non-pregnant women* | *Pregnant women* |
|---|---|---|
| Thyroid size | Normal | Enlarged by 70 % |
| Protein bound iodine | 276–630 nmol/litre | 552–1024 nmol/litre |
| Basal metabolic rate | −15 %–+15 % | +15 %–+30 % |
| $T_3$ resin uptake | 11–18 % | 5–10 % |
| Reverse triiodothyronine | 0.4 micrograms/litre | 0.54 micrograms/litre |

|  |  | *Trimester of pregnancy* | | |
|---|---|---|---|---|
|  |  | *First* | *Second* | *Third* |
| Triiodothyronine | 1.3–3.5 nmol/litre | 1.9–4.3 | 2.2–4.8 | 2.2–4.3 |
| Thyroxine | 56–150 nmol/litre | 89–217 | 100–228 | 96–227 |
| $T_3$ uptake | 83–121 % | 109–142 | 122–150 | 124–156 |
| Free thyroxine index | 55–145 | 75–168 | 77–163 | 70–160 |
| Thyroxine binding globulin | 6–18 mg/litre | 10–26 | 14–35 | 15–37 |
| Thyroid stimulating hormone | 1.0–3.2 mu/litre | 2.9 | 2.6 | 2.1 |

When the diagnosis of thyrotoxicosis is suspected but difficult to confirm biochemically, an increase in TSH in response to 200 micrograms of thyrotrophin releasing hormone given intravenously may prove useful in excluding thyrotoxicosis.

Hypothyroidism may be confirmed by demonstrating an elevated serum TSH, but the assay must not cross-react with chorionic gonadotrophin.

# Hypothyroidism

Myxoedema is rarely associated with pregnancy as its onset is usually postmenopausal or it is associated with loss of libido and menorrhagia which may impair fertility. The disease is four times commoner in women than men and multipara are especially at risk.

Overt hypothyroidism is characterized by mental and physical sluggishness, intolerance of cold, constipation and gain in weight. The patient has a characteristic appearance with a hoarse voice and dry skin. There is a malar flush which is typical of myxoedema and the hair is dry and brittle and tends to come out easily.

A perceptible delay in the relaxation of tendon jerks is characteristic of the disease. This symptom disappears rapidly with adequate treatment. Associated neurological problems include carpal tunnel syndrome, polyneuritis and myopathy. However, a detailed physical examination is of limited help in establishing the diagnosis as mild cases may lack any clinical changes.

Untreated hypothyroidism reduces fertility and is associated with a high fetal wastage and probably developmental abnormalities. The significance of very mild degrees of thyroid failure are uncertain in pregnancy.

## Investigation

Serum TSH is usually above 20 mIU/litre and associated with a low $T_3$ and FTI. A more moderate elevation is seen in patients without clinical evidence of hypothyroidism.

## Treatment

0.1 mg to 0.2 mg of thyroxine daily should be continued throughout pregnancy. The dose must be adequate to achieve euthyroidism, which is confirmed biochemically by a return of the serum TSH level to normal. The TSH level must be monitored on a monthly basis throughout the pregnancy.

Occasionally patients with untreated hypothyroidism conceive and complete their pregnancy successfully. They have an increased rate of stillbirth and although the offspring are often normal there is an increased incidence of physical and mental abnormalities. If the mother has particularly high levels of TSH and thyrotrophin releasing hormone, the baby is rarely at risk of developing neonatal thyrotoxicosis.

## Hyperthyroidism

Hyperthyroidism or thyrotoxicosis may be due to:

1. Diffuse hyperplasia and hypertrophy (Graves' Disease).
2. Hyperactive or 'toxic' nodules of the thyroid gland.
3. A 'silent' thyroiditis.
4. Increased placental thyrotrophin production in trophoblastic disease.
5. 'Struma ovarii' which is an ovarian teratoma which secretes TSH.

Thyrotoxicosis complicates 2 in a 1000 pregnancies. It is usually due to Graves' disease, but its clinical features are the same, regardless of cause. The disease onset is usually gradual but it can be dramatic and florid. There is usually weight loss despite a good appetite. The patient becomes easily fatigued, sweats and dislikes warm rooms. She may complain of palpitations, dyspnoea and even angina. On examination, the patient will have sinus tachycardia or atrial fibrillation with a collapsing pulse and sometimes evidence of cardiac failure. Diarrhoea and emotional lability are common. Perhaps the most characteristic signs are prominence of the eyes (exophthalmos) with lid retraction, lid lag, proptosis and often an ophthalmoplegia.

## Investigation

Generally a serum $T_4$ assay, preferably with reference to its binding proteins is all that is necessary to confirm or refute the diagnosis of thyrotoxicosis. Serum $T_3$ may help in difficult cases and where doubt remains, a TRH test may be of value. There is a low basal secretion of TSH and the response to TRH will be blunted or negative.

Long-acting thyroid stimulator–protector antibodies in the maternal blood in quantities of more than 20 units accurately predict the subsequent development of neonatal thyrotoxicosis.

## Treatment

Untreated thyrotoxicosis in pregnancy results in a high incidence of abortion, perinatal death and prematurity. The choice of treatment lies between surgery and medical therapy, as radioactive iodine is absolutely contraindicated. The choice is largely personal as there are no controlled trials to indicate which is the best form of treatment.

**Table 6.3**  Adverse effects of therapy in hyperthyroidism

| Medical treatment | Surgical treatment |
|---|---|
| 1. Failed treatment due to:<br>  i. Drug reaction<br>  ii. Poor compliance<br>2. Carbimazole may cause:<br>  i. Scalp defects<br>  ii. Aplasia cutis<br>3. Carbimazole is secreted in breast milk<br>4. Fetal hypothyroidism | 1. Anaesthetic risk<br>2. Hypoparathyroidism<br>3. Recurrent laryngeal nerve palsy |

### Medical treatment

There are two drugs which may be used.

1. Propylthiouracil.
2. Carbimazole or its active metabolite methimazole.

Propylthiouracil has distinct advantages over carbimazole. It crosses the placenta in smaller quantities and prevents the conversion of $T_4$ to $T_3$ which may speed the control of thyrotoxicosis. It is not concentrated in breast milk and only trivial doses will be received by the newborn infant. 100–150 mg of propylthiouracil are taken 8 hourly and the dose is reviewed monthly. The dose is gradually reduced so that the mother is euthyroid or mildly hyperthyroid. At no stage should the mother become hypothyroid; this is best recognized by following the serum TSH. However, if this does occur she must be given thyroxine. If carbimazole is used to control hyperthyroidism the initial dose should be 15 mg orally every 8 hours.

As thyroxine fails to cross the placenta to any extent there is no rationale for giving thyroxine to mothers receiving antithyroid drugs. Conversely, if a woman is well controlled but has a high long-acting thyroid stimulator – protector antibody titre there may be a place for carbimazole and thyroxine to suppress fetal hyperthyroidism while maintaining maternal euthyroidism. The effect of such treatment can be monitored by means of the fetal heart rate.

The current view that antithyroid drug treatment has no adverse effect on fetal development, has not passed unchallenged in many European centres, where women on antithyroid medication also receive oral contraceptives. There is little evidence to support the view that they cause central nervous abnormalities and long-term assessment of children exposed to carbimazole *in utero* has revealed no intellectual impairment.

Propranolol and other $\beta$ blockers control the symptoms of hyperthyroidism but do not alter the underlying metabolic abnormalities. Early experience with propranolol suggested a poor fetal outcome, but subsequent controlled studies testify to their safety although growth retardation is a common finding. Their long-term use in hyperthyroidism during pregnancy cannot be justified.

**Surgical treatment**

Failure of the patient to comply with medical treatment is an indication for surgery, as is failure to control the disease with moderate doses of antithyroid drugs. Surgical intervention is also of value when the patient has had a toxic reaction to antithyroid drugs. Surgery is mandatory when there is tracheal compression due to thyroid enlargement.

Subtotal thyroidectomy is traditionally performed in the second trimester. Preoperative preparations include the use of antithyroid drugs and propranolol to render the patient euthyroid. Potassium iodide is probably best avoided because of its tendency to produce a fetal goitre. Postoperatively the expectant mother should receive thyroxine replacement if the serum TSH level rises.

# Effect of thyrotoxicosis on the neonate

Most patients with Graves' disease have a specific autoimmune antibody–long-acting thyroid stimulator protector (LATS protector). Neonatal thyrotoxicosis is believed to result from its placental transfer and is seen in up to 10 per cent of babies born to mothers with a history of Graves' disease.

**Table 6.4**  Prediction of neonatal thyrotoxicosis

| Maternal features | Fetal features |
|---|---|
| 1. Pretibial myxoedema | 1. Fetal hyperkinesia |
| 2. Exophthalmos | 2. Fetal tachycardia |
| 3. Elevated levels of maternal thyroid stimulating immunoglobulins | |

The syndrome may be recognized by the small size of the baby and the presence of exophthalmos, a goitre, hypermetabolism, tachycardia and cardiac failure. At birth, the neonate can be euthyroid if the mother has received antithyroid drugs, as these cross the placenta. However, within 7 days of birth their effect will be ended and neonatal thyrotoxicosis may develop.

The condition carries a mortality as high as 16 per cent but it can be controlled with carbimazole which will need to be given for 3 months. During this time TSH, $T_4$ and $T_3$ levels should be monitored.

## Accidental use of radio-iodine during pregnancy

The mother should be given normal iodine and put on adequate replacement therapy. If the exposure occurs during the first 9 weeks, no abnormalities have been reported. The fetal thyroid begins synthesis of its hormones between the 9th and 12th weeks, after which radio-iodine can cause fetal hypothyroidism. Replacement therapy given to the mother at this time will not cross the placenta and is of no benefit to the fetus.

# Postpartum thyroiditis

In this syndrome, which is now recognized more frequently than in the past, a goitre and symptoms of hypothyroidism develop in the puerperium. The condition has been attributed to the sudden cessation of the immunological tolerance which characterizes pregnancy, in a person who is susceptible to autoimmune diseases. The condition is self-limiting and recovery occurs after a few months.

## Investigation

There is biochemical evidence of mild hypothyroidism and the thyroid antibody screen is usually positive.

## Treatment

Patients with significant symptoms should receive thyroxine for several months. It is then withdrawn and thyroid function reassessed.

# Thyroiditis

Subacute thyroiditis and chronic lymphocytic or Hashimoto's thyroiditis rarely complicate pregnancy. The former causes painful swelling of the gland and is associated with mild hyperthyroidism and a fever which lasts for several weeks. The tenderness and swelling of the thyroid gland will resolve over 4 months but occasionally the course is chronic and lasts much longer. In Hashimoto's thyroiditis there is a painless goitre associated with hypothyroidism and the condition is clearly associated with other autoimmune diseases.

## Investigation

In subacute thyroiditis the erythrocyte sedimentation rate (ESR) may exceed 100 mm/hour and low titres of thyroid antibodies may be found. Confirmation of the diagnosis can be difficult as radioactive iodine uptake tests are contraindicated. Thyroid antibodies are also found in Hashimoto's disease. Antibodies are directed against thyroglobulin, thyroid colloid and thyroid microsomes.

## Treatment

Treatment of subacute thyroiditis with steroids is highly effective and relatively safe. Less effective methods include the use of antithyroid drugs such as 30 mg carbimazole daily for 2 to 3 weeks or suppression with thyroxine. In Hashimoto's thyroiditis treatment with thyroxine is mandatory even if the thyroid function appears normal.

# Solitary thyroid nodules

Ten per cent of solitary masses in the thyroid gland are neoplastic. Unfortunately thyroid scans cannot be performed in pregnancy. After thyroid function tests have excluded a toxic adenoma and a thyroid antibody screen has ruled out a localized area of thyroiditis, a thyroid ultrasound examination should be carried out to discover whether the nodule is cystic or solid. Cystic lesions less than 4 cm in diameter are rarely malignant, but about a quarter of solid lesions are malignant. Solid lesions should be biopsied or surgically removed.

# Carcinoma of the thyroid gland

Although rare in pregnancy it should be considered in every patient with a goitre. The tumour must be removed without regard to the pregnancy. A previous history of carcinoma of this gland is not a contraindication to pregnancy and pregnancy does not adversely affect prognosis. If the patient is on suppressive therapy with thyroxine this should be continued through any subsequent pregnancy and careful watch kept for any evidence of recurrence.

## *Adrenal disorders*

There are physiological changes in adrenal function which occur during pregnancy.

**Table 6.5**  Changes in adrenocortical function during pregnancy

| | |
|---|---|
| 1. | Plasma cortisol levels double during the last two trimesters |
| 2. | Most of the cortisol is physiologically inactive as there is a simultaneous rise in corticosteroid binding globulin |
| 3. | There is a rise in free plasma cortisol during the last trimester |
| 4. | The circadian rhythm is preserved but the late night fall in free cortisol is less during pregnancy |
| 5. | Plasma aldosterone increases markedly from the sixteenth week of pregnancy |

# Adrenocortical insufficiency or Addison's disease

Chronic hypoadrenalism ranges from complete failure of hormone production to minor impairment of adrenal reserve capacity. Pigmentation of the skin may raise suspicion of the diagnosis. It is marked around the nipples, in the mouth and along skin creases or scars. Fatigue is a common but rather non-specific complaint. The patient may complain of anorexia, nausea, vomiting and weight loss. Many of these symptoms are common to pregnancy as well and this can make the diagnosis difficult. Hypotension in the erect posture is an important physical sign which can cause syncopal attacks.

Conception was rare before the advent of cortisone, and in those who did conceive, pregnancy often resulted in their death. The major causes of this were:

1. Electrolyte imbalance due to vomiting in the first trimester.
2. The stress of labour.
3. Opportunistic infections.

## Investigation

Cortisol production is usually reduced but may be at the lower end of the normal range under basal conditions. There is no incease, however, in response to stress because the adrenocortical reserve is reduced. This can be demonstrated by an impaired response to exogenous ACTH – the short tetracosactrin (Synacthen) test.

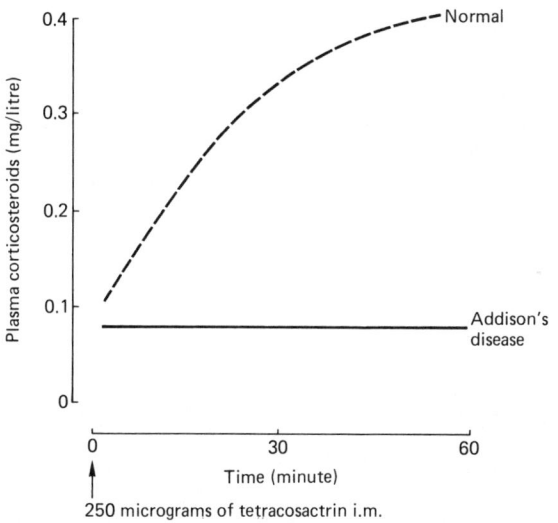

**Fig. 6.1** Short tetracosactrin test.

250 micrograms of tetracosactrin are given intramuscularly. Plasma cortisol is measured at 30 and 60 minutes. There is no increase in plasma cortisol in Addison's disease in response to the tetracosactrin.

## Treatment

In treated patients fertility is unimpaired. Treatment should continue in the same way as before the pregnancy. This may be with 37.5 mg of cortisone acetate or 30 mg of hydrocortisone daily; supplemented in some patients by a small dose of 9 α fluorohydrocortisone.

Special attention should be given to vomiting as additional intramuscular hydrocortisone is required as well as 0.05 mg to 0.1 mg daily of 9 α fluorohydrocortisone. Steroid therapy must be increased promptly to cover the stress of delivery. 100 mg of hydrocortisone is given intramuscularly on the evening before delivery and this is followed by 25 to 50 mg intramuscularly every 6 hours for the first 24 hours of the procedure and for the following day. The return to normal replacement dosage takes place over the next 8 to 10 days.

Children of mothers with Addison's disease tend to be small and are theoretically at risk of adrenocortical suppression at birth, but are otherwise normal.

# Cushing's syndrome

Cushing's syndrome results from excessive production of cortisol which may be due to overproduction of adrenocorticotrophin (ACTH). In most series spontaneous ACTH overproduction by the pituitary accounts for about 80 per cent of affected adults. Adrenocortical adenomas and carcinomas and the ectopic ACTH syndrome contribute equally to the remaining 20 per cent. The major clinical features of Cushing's syndrome are obesity, striae, hypertension and peripheral oedema, hirsutes, excessive bruising, muscle weakness, psychiatric disturbances, irregular menstruation, back pain and diabetes mellitus.

Amenorrhoea and sterility are common and the association of untreated Cushing's syndrome with pregnancy has been described in less than 50 cases. The frequency of abortion, prematurity and stillbirth is high and the fetus is at risk of adrenal insufficiency and fetal virilization.

Unless treatment is by pituitary ablation sexual function and fertility are restored. Women with a subtotal adrenalectomy or who are on replacement therapy must be monitored carefully throughout pregnancy as they may develop adrenal insufficiency.

**Table 6.6** Aetiology of Cushing's syndrome

| Cause | Serum levels ACTH | Cortisol |
|---|---|---|
| *ACTH excess* | | |
| *1. Cushing's disease* | | |
| Pituitary/hypothalamic disease | Increased | Increased |
| *2. Ectopic ACTH syndrome* | | |
| Malignant or benign non-endocrine hormone secreting tumour | Increased | Increased |
| *3. Iatrogenic* | | |
| ACTH administration for inflammatory or immunological disorders | Increased | Increased |
| *Cortisol Excess* | | |
| *1. Adrenal adenoma* | Suppressed | Increased |
| *2. Adrenal carcinoma* | Suppressed | Increased |
| *3. Iatrogenic* | | |
| Corticosteroids for inflammatory or immunological disorders | Suppressed | Cortisol or analogue increased |

## Investigation

*1. Tests of excess cortisol production:*

i. Urinary free cortisol.
ii. Urinary 17-oxogenic and 17-oxosteroids.
iii. Cortisol secretion rate.
iv. Plasma cortisol estimations at 0900 and 2400 hours may show loss of the normal circadian rhythm. A high level at midnight can be caused by stress such as hospital admission or even sampling technique.

*2. Tests of the cause of overproduction of cortisol:*

i. Plasma ACTH measurements at 0900 and 2400 hours will indicate whether the lesion is pituitary or adrenal in origin.
ii. The metyrapone test.
iii. Dexamethasone suppression tests.
iv. Skull X-rays with appropriate abdominal shielding.

The diagnosis of Cushing's syndrome in pregnancy is difficult as cortisol levels may be as high as those in some patients with adrenocortical hyperfunction.

## Treatment

Once the diagnosis of an adrenal tumour is made, surgical removal under appropriate steroid cover, should be performed. The contralateral atrophic gland will recover but trial reductions of the dose of hydrocortisone should be postponed until after delivery. In pituitary dependent disease, transfrontal hypophysectomy for tumours with suprasellar extension or transphenoidal hypophysectomy, should be considered. Replacement therapy will then be needed throughout pregnancy and labour, with a similar regime to that described for patients with Addison's disease.

# Congenital adrenal hyperplasia

This condition results from a defect in the biosynthesis of cortisol. The impaired cortisol production leads to an increased plasma ACTH level and adrenal hyperplasia. Precortisol metabolites accumulate and these are androgenic. Following surgical correction of fused labia and related defects the patient requires glucocorticoids such as prednisolone. The majority of the dose is given at night to maintain ACTH suppression on the lowest total dose eg. 2.5 mg prednisolone in the morning and 5 mg in the evening.

Despite adequate therapy, women tend to be short and have an android pelvis. They are fertile but often require delivery by Caesarian section.

# Primary aldosteronism (Conn's syndrome)

The association of Conn's syndrome with pregnancy is too rare to allow firm conclusions to be drawn regarding treatment and risks to the fetus.

During pregnancy, both plasma and urinary levels of aldosterone are increased, and this makes diagnosis difficult. Remission of the disorder can occur in pregnancy because the action of aldosterone is antagonized by progesterone.

# Phaeochromocytoma

The classical symptoms are intermittent episodes which begin with an aura which the patient may find difficult to describe but which consist of:

1. Epigastric fullness.
2. Apprehension.
3. Palpitations due to arrhythmias.
4. Excessive sweating and flushing.

These episodes are often associated with headache and may last for minutes to hours. Because the clinical features are intermittent and varied diagnosis on clinical grounds is unusual although suspicion may be high.

Phaeochromocytomas which become active during pregnancy are highly dangerous for mother and child. Untreated, maternal mortality may be as high as 50 per cent with a fetal mortality of 55 per cent. If the diagnosis is made before term, then the maternal mortality can be reduced with treatment, although the effect on the fetus is uncertain.

## Investigation

*All patients with paroxysmal or sustained hypertension should be screened for a phaeochromocytoma.*
There are also other groups who should be screened and these include:

1. Women with convulsions which resemble pre-eclamptic fits.
2. Women with symptoms suggestive of thyrotoxicosis, diabetes mellitus or an anxiety state.
3. Paroxysmal cardiac dysrhythmias.
4. Von Recklinghausen's disease.

The biochemical diagnosis is based on an increased catecholamine production. Urine is collected for three separate 24 hour periods and the metanephrine concentration is measured by spectrophotometry or gas chromatography. The vanoxymandelic acid (VMA) content is reliable if measured by a spectrophotometric method, but this is not so using a fluorimetric technique.

Radiological investigation and sampling from the adrenal veins should not be undertaken while the patient is pregnant.

## Treatment

In the first two trimesters surgical removal of the tumour is indicated. The risk of abortion is high. In the third trimester medical management with $\alpha$ adrenergic blockade (eg. with phenoxybenzamine) may control the hypertension and allow the fetus to reach maturity. Tachycardia in excess of 140 beats/minute and dysrhythmias may be controlled by cardioselective $\beta$ blockade with agents such as metoprolol, provided the patient has been adequately $\alpha$ blocked. Once the fetus is mature, delivery should be by Caesarian section.

# *Parathyroid disease*

## Primary hyperparathyroidism

This condition is most common in postmenopausal women and less than 50 cases associated with pregnancy have been reported. The patient may have recurrent renal calcium stones or bone disease. However, a substantial number of patients are asymptomatic and are detected on routine biochemical screening for hypercalcaemia.

In pregnancy, primary hyperparathyroidism leads to an increased incidence of stillbirths, premature labour and neonatal tetany.

## Investigation

**Table 6.7** Biochemical changes in hyperparathyroidism

| | |
|---|---|
| *Plasma* | |
| Calcium | Increased |
| Parathyroid hormone | Normal or increased |
| Phosphate | Decreased |
| Alkaline phosphatase | Normal or increased. *In pregnancy placental alkaline phosphatase may give a high reading on most autoanalysers* |
| *Urine* | |
| Calcium | Increased |
| Phosphate | Increased |

Preoperative localization of the tumour by immunoassay of venous blood sampled from various sites in the neck may be useful.

## Treatment

Patients with severe disease, in whom the calcium is greater than 3.0 mmol/litre require parathyroidectomy during the first two trimesters. During the third trimester it may be possible to delay surgery until early delivery of the fetus is accomplished at 36 weeks.

In mild cases with normal renal function, it is probably best to allow pregnancy and delivery to proceed normally. However, in all cases, tetany in the premature neonate will require vigorous treatment.

# Hypoparathyroidism

In the absence of parathyroid hormone, the plasma calcium falls to about 1.25 mmol/litre. Neuromuscular function is impaired and the patient develops tetany. Positive Trousseau's and Chvostek's signs may be elicited. Occasionally epilepsy is the presenting feature. Probably the most distressing feature is systemic candidiasis.

## Investigation

Biochemically the disease is characterized by:

1. An unmeasurable plasma parathyroid hormone.
2. A low serum calcium.
3. A high serum phosphate.

## Treatment

1–2 mg (40–80 000 units) of vitamin D daily have been successfully used to treat this condition. However, it is slow in its onset of action and may cause prolonged hypercalcaemia. 1 $\alpha$ hydroxycholecalciferol in doses of 1–2 micrograms/day or 0.5–2.0 micrograms/day of 1, 25 dihydroxycholecalciferol have been used to control the plasma calcium and phosphate. They have the advantage of rapid action and short half-life. They are the drugs of choice in pregnancy and provided there is good control of maternal hypoparathyroidism fetal development appears to be normal.

# Further reading

Burr, W.A. (1981). Thyroid disease. *Clinics in Obstetrics and Gynaecology* **8**, 341.

Jacobs, H.S. (1984). *Prolactinomas and Pregnancy*. MTP Press, Lancaster.

Montgomery, D.A.D. and Harley, J.M.G. (1977). Endocrine disorders. *Clinics in Obstetrics and Gynaecology* **4**, 339.

Pekonen, F. and Lamberg, B.A. (1978). Thyrotoxicosis during pregnancy. *Annales Chirurgiae et Gynaecologiae* **67**, 165.

Ramsay, I. (1980). Thyroid disease in pregnancy. *Hospital Update* **6**, 685.

Shearman, R.P. (1983). Inappropriate hyperprolactinaemia and secondary amenorrhoea. In *Progress in Obstetrics and Gynaecology*,Volume 3, 257. Edited by J. Studd. Churchill Livingstone, Edinburgh.

Turkalj, I., Brown, P. and Krupp, P. (1982). Surveillance of bromocriptine in pregnancy. *Journal of the American Medical Association* **247**, 1584.

# 7

# Diabetes and its control in pregnancy

At the beginning of the twentieth century maternal mortality in diabetic pregnancies was almost 30 per cent. However, this rapidly dropped to less than 10 per cent following the introduction of insulin and the treatment of ketoacidosis. The maternal mortality in diabetic pregnancies is now only slightly greater than in normal pregnancy. For many years perinatal mortality remained at 40 per cent, but the recent strict control of maternal blood sugar levels has reduced perinatal mortality to less than 5 per cent in specialist centres. This compares favourably with an overall perinatal mortality rate of less than 20 per cent in Great Britain. These results should encourage a diabetic woman to accept the considerable disruption that her pregnancy may cause, provided the medical team give adequate explanations and support.

## Classification of diabetes

There are several classifications of diabetes, but the following system is a useful working model.

1. *Chemical or asymptomatic diabetes.* The glucose tolerance test is abnormal but the patient has no clinical evidence of diabetes.
2. *Latent diabetes.* Under conditions of stress the glucose tolerance test is abnormal but it reverts to normal when the stress is removed. When pregnancy is the cause of the stress the disease is known as *Gestational diabetes.* Factors which increase the likelihood of the pregnant woman developing diabetes include:
   i. a family history of diabetes in first degree relatives;
   ii. a previous baby weighing more than 4.5 kg;
   iii. persistent glycosuria;
   iv. obesity with a weight greater than 90 kg. or 20 per cent above the ideal body weight;
   v. a previous unexplained perinatal death;

  vi. latent diabetes seen during a previous illness;
 vii. an abnormal obstetric history with recurrent miscarriage;
viii. previous unexplained congenital abnormality;
  ix. polyhydramnios.
   x. hypertension.
Of these factors the first four are probably the most significant risk factors.

  **3.** *Frank diabetes.* An abnormal glucose tolerance test associated with signs and symptoms of diabetes.

**Table 7.1** Priscilla White's classification of diabetes in pregnancy

| Class | Characteristics |
| --- | --- |
| A | Chemical diabetes |
| B | Duration less than 10 years<br>Onset after the age of 20 years<br>No complications |
| C | Duration of 10–19 years<br>Onset between age of 10 and 19 years<br>No complications |
| D | Duration of more than 20 years<br>Onset before the age of 10 years<br>Benign retinopathy |
| E | Calcified pelvic vessels |
| F | Diabetic nephropathy |
| R | Proliferative retinopathy |
| G | Multiple failed pregnancies |
| H | Heart disease |
| I | Renal transplant |

In 1942 Priscilla White proposed a classification of diabetes in pregnancy which related the duration, severity and treatment of diabetes in the pregnant state to prognosis. It was modified in 1965. Although it allows comparisons between different centres, it is of no value in determining management during pregnancy.

## Normal maternal and fetal carbohydrate metabolism

Pregnancy is a state of insulin resistance where normal glucose homeostasis is maintained by an increased rate of insulin secretion. Insulin resistance is due to a number of factors which includes loss of glucose to the fetus and possibly the urine. In addition, insulin is degraded by the placenta and adrenal steroid production is increased. The growth hormone-like effect of human chorionic somatomammotrophin increases insulin resistance. This challenge to the pancreas may lead to gestational diabetes in women with potential diabetes.

**Table 7.2** Hormonal effects of glucose metabolism and insulin secretion during pregnancy

| Hormone | Actions |
| --- | --- |
| Oestradiol | ↑ insulin secretion<br>↓ gluconeogenesis |
| Progesterone | ↑ insulin secretion<br>↓ glucagon secretion |
| Human placental lactogen | ↑ blood glucose<br>Blocks effect of oestradiol and progesterone |

In normal pregnancy of 10 weeks gestation the fasting blood glucose falls to a significantly lower level than in the non-pregnant patient and then remains relatively unchanged throughout the rest of the pregnancy. Fasting blood sugar levels are therefore normally lower in pregnancy (3.4–4.5 mmol/litre). As pregnancy advances, there is a slight increase in the postprandial blood glucose level and the peak plasma glucose is progressively delayed towards the end of pregnancy. This delay is associated with a progressive increase in the peak insulin concentration.

During pregnancy the mean plasma glucose remains below 5.6 mmol/litre except during the hour after a meal and although it rises in late pregnancy it is only by 0.2 mmol/litre. This is associated with an increase in plasma insulin levels as a result of tissue resistance to insulin. If the pancreas is unable to produce sufficient insulin, chemical diabetes results.

Fetal energy requirements are met primarily by glucose which crosses the placenta by facilitated diffusion. In diabetes the raised plasma glucose in the mother is reflected by a similar rise in the fetus. This stimulates hyperplasia of the islets of Langerhans and this causes hyperinsulinism, hypoglycaemia and excessive lipogenesis which leads to fetal macrosomia (a large body). There is a clear relationship between the average maternal blood sugars during the last trimester and the amount of subcutaneous fat in the neonate as assessed by skin fold thickness measurements. Fetal size increases during the last trimester and control of maternal plasma glucose is especially important from the thirtieth week of gestation.

# Diagnosis of diabetes in pregnancy

## Single blood glucose levels

Single measurements may be used to identify patients at particular risk who are suitable for further testing. Glucose levels may be measured in the fasting state, after breakfast or after a glucose challenge. It is particularly important to do this in patients with a

**Table 7.3** Single blood glucose levels as risk factors with or without prior carbohydrate ingestion (Modified from Barden and Knowles, 1981)*

|  | Authors | | | | |
|---|---|---|---|---|---|
|  | Guttorm | Chen et al | O'Sullivan | Amankwah et al | Merkatz et al |
| Gestation | 12–16 weeks | | Any stage | 32–33 weeks | 24–28 weeks |
| Time | Fasting | Postprandial | Afternoon | | Fasting |
| Preparation | None | Breakfast | 50 g glucose | 50 g glucose | 75 g glucose |
| Sampling time | | 2 hour | 1 hour | 1 hour | 2 hour |
| Specimen | Venous plasma | Venous blood | Venous plasma | Venous plasma | Capillary blood |
| Positive test (mmol/litre) | ≥5 | >5.6 | ≥8.3 | >7.2 | >6.7 |
| Prevalence of diabetes identified by technique | 1.7% | 1.1% | 2.0% | 2.0% | 3.1% |

* There are a variety of techniques for selection of a single blood glucose level which is suggestive of diabetes. The criteria chosen by Chen et al are particularly helpful.

history of glycosuria or other risk factors. If the levels exceeds 5.6 mmol/litre, an oral glucose tolerance test should be performed.

## Oral glucose tolerance tests

**Table 7.4** Indications for an oral glucose tolerance test during pregnancy (Modifed from West, 1978)

| | | |
|---|---|---|
| *Maternal* | 1. | Two episodes of glycosuria in the fasted patient |
| | 2. | A high postprandial blood glucose |
| | 3. | Family history of diabetes in first degree relatives |
| | 4. | An obese woman with a body weight greater than 120 % ideal weight |
| *Obstetric* | 1. | Previous baby larger than 4.5 kg |
| | 2. | Previous unexplained perinatal death |
| | 3. | Previous gestational diabetes |
| | 4. | Recurrent abortion |

In normal pregnancy the oral glucose tolerance test is unchanged until the third trimester when there is often a small rise in blood sugar values, which remain within the normal range. To establish a diagnosis of diabetes a 75 g oral glucose tolerance test is currently used. In early pregnancy the glucose load may cause nausea and some consequently advocate an intravenous test.

The patient remains on a normal diet containing at least 150 g of carbohydrate for each of the 3 days preceding the test. No alcohol should be ingested after the previous evening meal. The test should be conducted in the morning after at least 8 but no more than 16 hours of fasting. Initially a fasting venous blood sample is taken and then 75 g glucose in 200–500 ml of flavoured water drunk in five minutes. Zero time is taken as the beginning of the drink and samples are withdrawn at 30 minute intervals for 2 hours. Values of blood glucose of 9.5 mmol/litre at 2 hours or a greater than 12.5 mmol/litre at any other time indicates diabetes in the non-pregnant woman.

The criteria recommended for diagnosis of abnormal glucose tolerance in pregnancy have varied among authors from minimal degrees of elevation of blood glucose to those levels used to diagnose established diabetes in non-pregnant women. In the same patient there are marked differences in glucose tolerance according to the duration of the pregnancy and in different pregnancies.

Recent attempts have been made to diagnose maternal diabetes in relation to perinatal outcome. A plasma glucose level of less than 1.7 mmol/litre in the neonate 2 hours after delivery is closely correlated with impaired glucose tolerance. Diabetes in pregnancy may be diagnosed when the area under a 50 g oral glucose tolerance test curve is greater than 43 SI units.

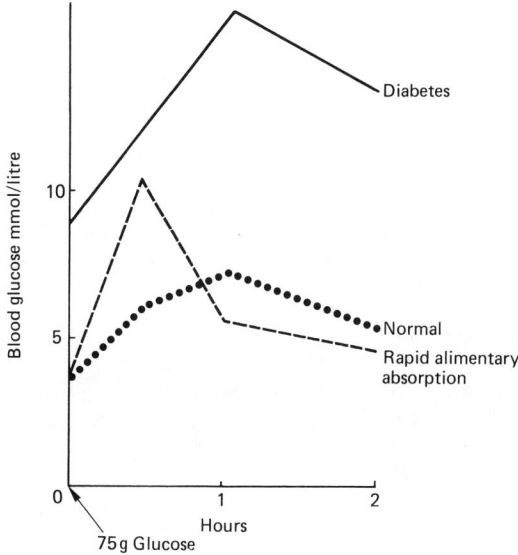

**Fig. 7.1** Glucose tolerance test in diabetes, rapid alimentary absorption and normal people.

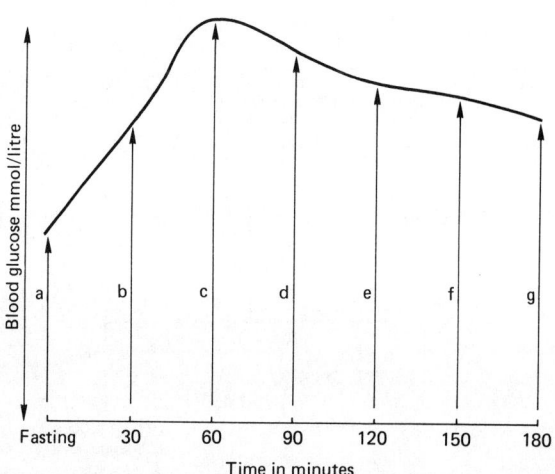

**Fig. 7.2** Method of calculating comparative areas for three hour GTTs. Area under curve = ½a + b + c + d + e + f + ½g (Modified from Friend, 1981).

## Intravenous glucose tolerance test

75 g of glucose is given intravenously over 30 minutes and then blood glucose measurements are done at 10 minute intervals for 1 hour. The shape of the slope of falling blood glucose indicates glucose tolerance. The rate of fall of glucose is referred to as the disappearance rate. In uncomplicated pregnancy, the disappearance rate of glucose has been shown to increase in the first trimester and fall below normal in the third trimester. The effect of pregnancy on intravenous glucose tolerance is uncertain and most centres rely on oral tests.

## Steroid provocative tests

In the past, cortisone or prednisone provocative tests were used to detect glucose intolerance during pregnancy. However, the results of various comparative studies have been conflicting and steroid challenge tests have lost their popularity.

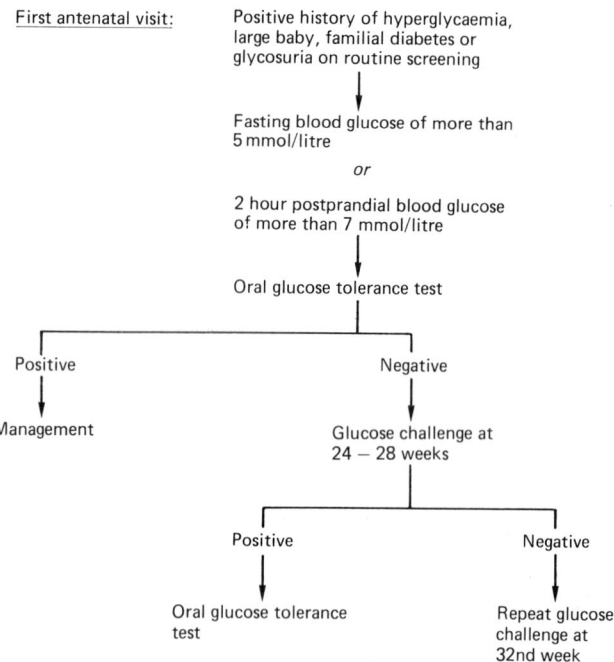

**Fig. 7.3**  Clinical protocol for detection and investigation of abnormal glucose tolerance in pregnancy (Modified from Barden and Knowles, 1981).

# Maternal complications associated with diabetic pregnancies

## Medical complications

Levels of control normally adequate for the non-pregnant woman are no longer acceptable in pregnancy where hypoglycaemia and ketosis effect the fetus adversely. Loss of diabetic control in the third trimester may contribute directly to fetal mortality.

In the past, diabetic women with renal, myocardial and retinal vascular disease were advised to have their pregnancies terminated. Diabetic nephropathy is a progressive disease found mostly in those patients with a history of insulin-dependent diabetes mellitus for more than 15 years. The syndrome is one of proteinuria, peripheral oedema and gradually increasing renal failure. Hypertension develops in a large number of patients and renal function deteriorates until chronic renal failure develops. The diagnosis of diabetic nephropathy in pregnancy is made on the basis of persistent proteinuria of greater than 400 mg /24 hours during the first trimester, in the absence of urinary tract infection. The amount of proteinuria often increases dramatically during the last trimester and results in nephrotic syndrome. The severity of the proteinuria does not appear to affect maternal or fetal outcome but it is linked to hypertension and its distinction from eclampsia is often impossible.

Information about coronary artery disease during pregnancy in diabetics is sparse. Women over 30, or with an onset of diabetes prior to the age of ten, should have an electrocardiogram and if they are anxious to continue the pregnancy, they must take adequate rest and serial ECGs should be obtained. If cardiac failure develops rest,

**Table 7.5** Diabetic retinopathy

---

1. *Non-proliferative background retinopathy*
    i. Microaneurysms
    ii. Dot and blot haemorrhages
    iii. Hard exudates (yellow irregular)
    iv. Arteriolar abnormalities
    v. Arteriovenous nipping
    vi. Retinal oedema

2. *Preproliferative retinopathy (likely to progress to neovasularization)*
    i. Soft exudates
    ii. Venous abnormalities
    iii. Intraretinal microvascular abnormalities
    iv. Extensive dot and blot haemorrhages

3. *Proliferative retinopathy*
    i. Neovascularization either at the disc or elsewhere
    ii. Preretinal haemorrhage
    iii. Vitreous haemorrhage
    iv. Retinal detachment

---

sodium and fluid retention, possibly digoxin and diuretics are required.

The most common form of vascular disease in diabetes is retinopathy the natural history of which is controversial. Pregnancy is associated with a deterioration of preproliferative or proliferative retinopathy and most physicians have advised avoidance or termination of pregnancy. Deterioration of retinopathy may be prevented by previous therapy with laser photocoagulation. Severe florid disc neovascularization in the first trimester requires immediate panretinal photocoagulation and therapeutic abortion should be recommended. Pregnancy may be attempted later during a remission. Women with active proliferative retinopathy who complete their pregnancy should undergo delivery by Caesarian section to prevent rupture of the vessels.

The diabetic mother is likely to have obstetric complications which include:

1. Polyhydramnios – the amount of liquor may be reduced by strict control of the diabetes.
2. Pre-eclampsia.
3. Infection – especially of the urinary tract and also monilial vaginitis, both of which respond to conventional therapy.
4. Premature labour.
5. Fetal abnormalities.

## Fetal complications in diabetic pregnancies

Fetal mortality is increased due to abnormalities, intra-uterine death, premature delivery and during the perinatal period from respiratory distress syndrome, hypoglycaemia and congenital defects especially of the nervous and cardiovascular systems. The risk of fetal death is particularly high during the last 6 weeks of the pregnancy. Intensive treatment of maternal diabetes improves fetal survival, although the incidence of fetal abnormalities may not be affected. Improved control of maternal diabetes coupled with later delivery lessens the incidence of respiratory distress syndrome as a cause of neonatal death.

## Diabetic care before conception

Malformation of the heart and kidneys and sacral agenesis are the most common abnormalities found in the infants of diabetic mothers, so that the influence of diabetes on these structures must occur within the first seven weeks of pregnancy. The evidence suggests a metabolic rather than genetic aetiology. Since these abnormalities occur in the first trimester all diabetic pregnancies should be planned with the intention of maintaining strict diabetic control before conception. Indeed there is some evidence that hyperglycaemia will interfere with meiosis in the ovum.

# Antenatal management

The diabetic pregnant patient is best supervised by a combined obstetric and medical team. Patients fall into one of three main categories.

1. Those whose diabetes is diagnosed during pregnancy (gestational diabetes is a retrospective diagnosis).
2. Those with established diabetes of 10 years duration or less with mild or no complications.
3. Those with established diabetes for more than 10 years and those with serious renal or retinal damage.

In the first two groups the prospect of producing a live healthy infant after an uncomplicated pregnancy is good. Those in the third group often have a difficult pregnancy, despite good control of blood sugar.

## Surveillance of blood sugar

The aim should be normoglycaemia throughout the whole pregnancy – certainly from its diagnosis. Control is monitored by the following tests.

### Urine glucose

In pregnancy the diabetic is encouraged to test her urine four times a day before meals to coincide with preprandial blood glucose estimations. The bladder is first emptied and the second sample passed 15–20 minutes later is used for analysis. This method of control is unreliable and not recommended in pregnancy.

### Blood glucose

The need for rapid determination of blood glucose levels led to the introduction of a glucose oxidase impregnated stick with a colour indicator. Matching of the colour with a chart can lead to error. This has now been overcome by the use of reflectance meters. The majority of young diabetics prefer capillary blood sampling to urine testing when given the choice and this allows the patient to be closely involved with the regulation of her own diabetes and the fine adjustment of timing and dose of insulin. Capillary blood sampling can be performed three times daily.

With the introduction of such techniques it is now possible to keep patients out of hospital until admission is required for delivery. Previously patients were admitted at 32 weeks for monitoring.

## Glycosylated haemoglobin

In 1968 a glycosylated haemoglobin was identified in red cells. It is due to a modification of HbA to $HbA_1$ in the presence of hyperglycaemia. The amount of $HbA_1$ is directly proportional to the concentration of glucose within the red cell over a period of time. In normal non-pregnant women it accounts for 5.5–9.5 per cent of the total haemoglobin. The proportion is increased by three to four fold in poorly controlled diabetics. In pregnancy there is a significant reduction in the percentage of glycosylated haemoglobin by 20 weeks (Lind and Cheyne, 1979). The level recorded at the first antenatal visit will provide some guide to the level of control at the time of conception and embryonic development. Monthly samples enable a continuous assessment of control and may identify any dietary indiscretions by the patient.

## Ketonuria

The presence of ketones in urine which also contains glucose indicates accelerated ketogenesis and an acute lack of insulin. Ketonuria alone may be associated with starvation, vomiting or fever. The presence of ketones in pregnancy is closely associated with intellectual impairment of the child.

Pregnant diabetic mothers should be seen regularly in clinic. Their plasma glucose should be checked at 2 weekly intervals together with the urine for ketones. Ideally they should be provided with a meter for monitoring blood glucose at home and the aims of treatment explained carefully. The presence of hyperglycaemia and significant ketonuria at any time should be regarded as an indication for prompt admission to improve control.

**Table 7.6** Dietary and insulin modification in the presence of abnormal blood sugars

| *Example of a patient on actrapid and monotard insulin* | | | |
|---|---|---|---|
| *Time of elevated blood sugar* | | *Adjustment of diet and insulin* | |
| | | *Diet* | *Insulin* |
| | 0700 | — | p.m. monotard |
| *Insulin* at ——— | | | |
| 0800 hours | 1000 | Breakfast | a.m. actrapid |
| | 1200 | Elevenses | a.m. actrapid |
| | 1500 | Lunch | a.m. monotard |
| | 1800 | Mid afternoon Break | a.m. monotard |
| *Insulin* at ——— | | | |
| 1800 hours | 2200 | Tea | p.m. actrapid |
| | 0300 | Supper | p.m. monotard |

## Diet during pregnancy

To meet the nutritional needs of the fetus there must be an increase in all nutrients. There is disagreement on the question of maternal calorie intake and the restriction of dietary carbohydrate and fat in diabetic pregnancies. Some authorities recommend strict limitation of weight gain (White, 1971) and others only restrict calorie intake in obese pregnant diabetics (Pedersen, 1975). A major concern related to this question is the development of ketonuria which is associated with intellectual impairment (Berendes, 1975). It should not occur in the adequately fed pregnant mother. Calorie restriction cannot be advocated as the main treatment of the obese pregnant diabetic, but adequate insulin must be provided. Patients should receive 150 g to 200 g of carbohydrate daily and ketonuria treated with 20 g of additional carbohydrate at the three main meals.

## Oral hypoglycaemic agents

There is little place for the use of these agents in diabetes during pregnancy, although some have advocated their use in insulin independent diabetes without evidence of ketosis (Notelovitz, 1974). These patients, if untreated, have high perinatal mortality. It is possible to obtain adequate control of blood sugar with 250 mg of chlorpropamide or 1.5 g of tolbutamide daily in mild diabetes. However, these agents cross the placenta and may cause neonatal hypoglycaemia if they are not stopped 48 hours prior to delivery. There is limited experience with the use of metformin during the latter part of pregnancy and it cannot be recommended.

## Insulin

The aim of treatment is to keep the 2 to 3 hour postprandial plasma glucose below 7.2 mmol at home and below 6.0 mmol when resting in hospital. Repeated and severe hypoglycaemia must be avoided. The pregnant diabetic should maintain, as far as possible, a constant routine in the method, timing and site for insulin injection; always keeping the same site for injection at a particular time of day. This reduces factors which alter the rate of absorption of the insulin.

The most flexible and acceptable regimen involves a twice daily injection of mixture of short (soluble or actrapid) and medium acting insulins, (eg. Isophane, NPH, or Leo Retard). The use of purified or monocomponent insulins is preferred. Adjustment of one of these four doses together with a contribution from endogenous insulin allows adequate control. A further, third injection of short-acting insulin is preferable to the use of intermediate or long-acting single dose insulin regimes. Insulin requirements increase during pregnancy especially after 30–32 weeks gestation and may at 40 weeks be twice the requirements prior to conception.

Free maternal insulin does not cross the placenta but maternal insulin antibodies probably do and may damage fetal $\beta$ islet cells, predisposing to diabetes in later life. Antibody formation is less common with highly purified and human insulins which are to be preferred in young women.

## Effect of diabetes on obstetric measurements

The current trend is away from endocrine monitoring during pregnancy and in favour of ultrasound biometry in combination with cardiotocography. If endocrine tests are used it should be remembered that human placental lactogen (HPL) levels are high but only marginally above the normal range in diabetic pregnancies. *Falling insulin requirements are indicative of a decrease in fetal growth rate and may precede intra-uterine death.*

## Diabetic management during delivery

If well controlled, delivery is now usually timed for 40 weeks. Careful assessment of the mode of delivery is required and 'trials of labour' are best avoided in favour of elective Caesarian section. Diabetic pregnancy is one of the few remaining indications for measurement of the amniotic fluid lecithin/sphingomyelin ratio. However, its use has declined in response to improved maternal glucose control and neonatal intensive care. If the L:S ratio is to be used, it should be remembered that acceptable values tend to be 25 per cent above the commonly accepted indices of maturity.

Urgent delivery or the use of ritodrine or salbutamol to arrest premature labour, dramatically increases insulin requirements which should be given intravenously at rates as high as 30 units hourly, according to blood sugar levels. Lack of careful monitoring in this situation can lead to ketoacidosis. If dexamethasone is given to hasten fetal lung maturation diabetic control may be upset and hyper-glycaemia is best corrected by intravenous insulin infusion.

Until the day of planned induction of labour, diet and insulin are taken as usual. On the day of delivery an infusion of 1 litre of 5 per cent dextrose 6 hourly is started. Insulin is best given continuously by an infusion pump at an initial rate of 1–2 units/hour of actrapid insulin. If the blood sugar exceeds 8 mmol/litre, the infusion rate should be 4 units hourly with 1–2 hourly checks on the blood glucose. The insulin infusion is stopped immediately on delivery and subcutaneous insulin resumed according to need. The dose is similar to the pre-pregnancy requirements. The 5 per cent dextrose drip should be maintained until the patient resumes feeding.

If a continuous infusion pump is not available insulin may be added to the infusion fluid or it may be given by intermittent subcutaneous injection, the dose being controlled by blood sugar estimations. After delivery the pre-pregnancy regime is started as soon as possible.

Six weeks after delivery mothers with gestational diabetes should undergo a further glucose tolerance test. In many the abnormality persists and some patients become permanently diabetic.

**Perinatal problems**

The potential complications include:

1. High birth weight.
2. Respiratory distress syndrome.
3. Hypoglycaemia.
4. Hypocalcaemia and tetany.
5. Hypomagnaesaemia.
6. Polycythaemia.
7. Hyperbilirubinaemia.
8. Infection.

With better control, gross anatomical abnormalities are unusual, although some infants are still obese and mildly oedematous. Neonatal hypoglycaemia is the most serious complication of maternal diabetes and if the capillary blood glucose falls below 1.7 mmol/litre intravenous glucose must be given. Oral feeding is started within 2 or 3 hours of delivery and frequent glucose analyses are made.

# Further reading

Friend, J.R. (1981). Diabetes. *Clinics in Obstetrics and Gynaecology* **8**, 353.

Ireland, J.T., Thomson, W.S.T. and Williamson J. (1979). *Diabetes Today. A Handbook For the Clinical Team.* H.M. and M. Publishers, Aylesbury.

Kitzmiller, J.L., Aiello, L.M., Kaldany A. and Younger, M.D. (1981). Diabetic vascular disease complicating pregnancy. *Clinical Obstetrics and Gynecology* **24**, 107.

Oakley, W.G., Pyke, D.A. and Taylor, K.W. (1978). *Diabetes and its Management.* Oxford University Press, Oxford.

# References

Amankwah, K.S., Prentice, R.L. and Fleury, F.J., (1977). The incidence of gestational diabetes. *Obstetrics and Gynecology* **49**, 497.

Barden, T.P. and Knowles, H.C. (1981). Diagnosis of diabetes in pregnancy. *Clinics in Obstetrics and Gynaecology* **4**, 334.

Berendes, H.W. (1975). In *Early Diabetes in Early Life.* Edited by

Camerini-Davalds, R.A. and Cole, H.S. Academic Press, New York.

Chen, W, Palav, A. and Tricomi, V. (1972). Screening for diabetes in a perinatal clinic. *Obstetrics and Gynecology* **40**, 567.

Gabbe, S.G. and Quilligan, E.J., (1981). General obstetric management of the diabetic pregnancy. *Clinical Obstetrics and Gynecology* **24**, 91.

Guttorm, E. (1975). Practical screening for diabetic mellitus in pregnant women. In *Carbohydrate Metabolism in Pregnancy and Newborn*. Edited by Sutherland, H.W. Churchill Livingstone, London.

Knopp, R.H., Childs, M.T. and Warth, M.R., (1979). Dietary management of the pregnant diabetic. *Current Concepts in Nutrition* **8**, 119.

Lind, T. and Cheyne, G.A. (1979). Effect of normal pregnancy upon the glycosylated haemoglobins. *British Journal of Obstetrics and Gynaecology* **86**, 210.

Merkatz, I.R., Uchon, M.A., Yamashita, T.S. and Houser, H.B. (1980). A pilot community-based screening programme for gestational diabetes. *Diabetes Care* **3**, 453.

Montgomery, D.A.D. and Harley, J.M.G. (1977). Endocrine disorders. *Clinics in Obstetrics and Gynaecology* **4**, 339.

Notelovitz, M. (1974). Oral hypoglycaemic therapy in diabetic pregnancies. *Lancet* **2**, 902.

O'Sullivan, J.B., Mahan, C.M., Charles, D. and Dandrow, R.V. (1973). Screening criteria for high risk gestational diabetic patients. *American Journal of Obstetrics and Gynecology.* **116**, 895.

Pendersen, J. (1975). In *Early Diabetes in Early Life*. Edited by Camerini-Davalos, R.A. and Cole, H.S. Academic Press, New York.

West, T.E.T. (1980). Problems in Pregnancy Part 1: Diabetic Pregnancy. *Hospital Update* **6**, 585.

White, P. (1942). Pregnancy complicating diabetes. *American Journal of Medicine* **7**, 609.

White, P. (1971) In *Joslin's Diabetes Mellitus*. Edited by Marble, A., White, P., Bradley, R.F. and Krall. L.F. Lea and Febiger, Philadelphia.

# 8

# Gastro-intestinal disease in pregnancy

Gastro-oesophageal reflux and constipation are the most common gastro-intestinal symptoms in pregnancy due to the generalized relaxation of tone and decreased motility of smooth muscle. Less important are changes in intra-abdominal pressure and configuration as a result of the enlarging uterus.

## Hiatus hernia and pregnancy heartburn

'Heart-burn' occurs in about two thirds of pregnancies and is probably due to gastro-oesophageal reflux. It is not always associated with a hiatus hernia. Reflux of bile and acid from the stomach to the oesophagus occurs perhaps through an incompetent cardio-oesophageal sphincter. Manometric studies have shown that the lower oesophageal sphincter pressure is reduced in pregnancy.

### Investigation

Unless symptoms are severe, investigation is not indicated. If it becomes necessary, endoscopy is preferable to radiological examination.

### Treatment

This should include simple mechanical measures aimed at preventing acid and bile reflux. Such measures include the avoidance of stooping and bending at the waist and wearing tight garments. Oesophageal clearance at night is aided by raising the head of the bed.

Alginates, such as Gastrocote and Gaviscon are designed to float over gastric contents. Both agents also contain antacids which neutralize the low pH of gastric contents. Published experience of these agents in pregnancy is limited due to a reluctance to prescribe or take medicines during pregnancy, and the knowledge that symptoms will remit spontaneously in the puerperium. They are not, however, contraindicated in pregnancy. If the symptoms are due to bile reflux, dilute hydrochloric acid may be of value.

In severe cases which are resistant to the above measures, European experience with the anti-cholinesterase pyridostigmine (60 mg once daily) has shown it to be effective in providing symptomatic relief. The agent produced no adverse effects in the mother or fetus, but was not used in the last month of pregnancy.

# Peptic ulcer

Oestrogens produce a beneficial effect on the symptoms and healing of duodenal ulcers in men. The majority of women with peptic ulcers who become pregnant tend to improve; this may be because of a reduced secretion of gastric acid in the second trimester of pregnancy. The improvement does not persist after delivery.

## Investigations

Dyspepsia in pregnant women may be safely investigated by endoscopy rather than radiological investigations. It will also provide an opportunity to biopsy a gastric ulcer to exclude malignancy.

## Treatment

Although antacids provide symptomatic relief; they are required in large doses to heal ulcers (30 mls at 1 and 3 hours after meals and at bedtime; a total of 210 mls daily). However, $H_2$ receptor antagonists such as cimetidine and ranitidine, effectively heal peptic ulcers, but their effects on the fetus have not been investigated and the manufacturers do not recommend their routine use.

# Coeliac disease

This originally referred to a disease of children characterized by steatorrhoea, diarrhoea and malnutrition with stunting of growth and characteristic changes in the gastro-intestinal mucosa which recover with gluten restriction. About three-quarters of adult patients with steatorrhoea have no history of childhood illness and present with anaemia or lassitude. Folic acid deficiency is almost invariable and is the most common cause of anaemia; transient glossitis may be a symptom.

Infertility and spontaneous abortion is found in patients with untreated coeliac disease. This was first reported in the early 1970s and successful pregnancy occurred when patients were put on a gluten free diet.

## Investigations

A jejunal biopsy is a diagnostic procedure which will confirm or refute the presence of coeliac disease. Subtotal villous atrophy is characteristic of the disease. Histology reveals three main points:

1. A damaged surface epithelium.
2. The crypts are long and the lamina propria is infiltrated with chronic inflammatory cells.
3. The basement membrane is frequently thickened.

## Treatment

Lifelong dietary gluten restriction is essential. Relapse is frequent, fertility is improved, nutrition is maintained and there is some evidence that it prevents the development of malignancy. A gluten free diet means withdrawal of wheat, rye, barley, oats and all products made from their flour. Gluten free products are available on prescription for patients with coeliac disease and a list of gluten free foods can be obtained from The Coeliac Society (PO Box 181, London, NW2 2QY).

Failure to respond to dietary treatment means that corticosteroids may be required. Prednisolone in divided doses up to a total of 60 mg a day may be needed initially, but should be reduced to a minimum later.

Ogborn (1975) reported the pregnancies of 25 patients with coeliac disease. They had 38 pregnancies before starting a gluten free diet and 22 after. There was a 21 per cent spontaneous abortion rate in the untreated patients which may have been due to low serum folate levels. Treatment with a gluten free diet and folic acid replacement results in successful full term pregnancies. Treatment appears to have no effect on the gestational size of babies, 17 per cent of whom are small-for-dates.

## *Inflammatory bowel disease*

## Crohn's disease

Like syphylis and diabetes, Crohn's disease may present with protean clinical features so that diagnosis may remain obscure for some time. The clinical manifestations are due to obstruction and inflammation of the bowel and to systemic manifestations of chronic inflammation and malnutrition.

Some patients present with an acute illness indistinguishable from acute appendicitis or an appendix abscess while others have a history of chronic abdominal symptoms with pain, diarrhoea, ill health, weight loss and fever. On physical examination, malnutrition and anaemia with finger clubbing are common features. Abdominal examination may reveal signs of intestinal obstruction during acute episodes, whereas at other times there may be tenderness over the colon or a palpable mass, especially in the right iliac fossa. This may be associated with an abscess, resulting in psoas spasm and consequent flexion of the hip.

Anal or rectal lesions are common at some stages of the illness and there may be multiple anal fissures associated with fleshy oedematous skin tags. Perianal or ischiorectal abscesses can be very painful while indolent undermining ulceration may destroy the anal sphincter and cause faecal incontinence. Some patients have cutaneous lesions including erythema nodosum and pyoderma gangrenosa. About a third of patients have joint symptoms at some time, with the knee, ankle and wrist most commonly affected with swelling, pain and effusions. In 5 per cent of cases the patients also have ankylosing spondylitis.

## Investigation

In the non-pregnant state the diagnosis is often made by radiological examination. Where this is excluded, histological examination of biopsy material or surgically resected specimens, may show granulomata composed of epithelioid and giant cells of Langhans type and occasionally Schaumann bodies. The submucosa of narrowed areas will be thickened with proliferation of lymphoid tissue and oedema. All layers of the intestinal wall are inflamed and deep ulcers may penetrate the muscle coat to form internal and external fistulae.

## Treatment

Although surgery is still important, the correction of nutritional deficiencies and the use of drugs now make major contributions. Corticosteroids, sulphasalazine and even azathioprine may control acute exacerbations of the disease, but with the exception of sulphasalazine, their value in long-term suppression is limited. While surgery seldom cures the disease, it is an effective local treatment for an area of severe disease. The less widespread the disease, the lower the risk of recurrence. Overall the recurrence rate after most surgical procedures is about 50 per cent within 10 years.

It seems likely that women with Crohn's disease are subfertile. In a small unpublished study from South Wales 44 women with Crohn's disease were studied and 23 were aged between 16 and 35. Of the 14 women who became pregnant only 4 did so after their diagnosis was made. Difficulty in conception appears to be greater with Crohn's colitis than with small bowel disease and this may be due to Fallopian tube occlusion. Resection of the terminal ileum can lead to vitamin $B_{12}$ deficiency and this may also impair fertility.

Unless it is severe, Crohn's disease has no adverse effects on pregnancy. The frequency of abortion and stillbirth is no greater than in the general population. There appears to be no increased frequency of congenital abnormalities and the use of steroids or sulphasalazine should be continued through pregnancy, if required by the patient. A major concern with sulphasalazine is the development of kernicterus in the breast-fed neonate. However, only negligible amounts appear in breast milk and the main metabolite, sulphapyridine, only slightly displaces bilirubin from serum proteins.

Patients whose disease is inactive at conception appear to do well. Those who have had surgical resection of the disease appear to have the most favourable course and the majority of patients do not undergo a relapse. Patients with active disease at the time of conception have a variable course and some improve during the pregnancy. The outlook for patients who develop Crohn's disease during pregnancy is grim and may include maternal death. The majority of published cases report fetal death and a frequent need for surgical intervention. In all reported series there has been significant recurrence of disease in the puerperium and particularly in those who have not undergone surgery. Nevertheless prophylactic steroids in the puerperium are probably not indicated.

## Ulcerative colitis

Inflammation which is confined to the rectum (proctitis) usually presents with intermittent rectal bleeding as the only manifestation. Many patients are constipated but some have a normal bowel habit. When the inflammation is more extensive, the patient usually complains of diarrhoea and the passage of blood and mucus. If the whole of the colon is involved the stool may be liquid. There is an urgent desire to pass faeces and a marked increase in stool frequency. The condition may progress to toxic dilatation.

Various diseases are associated with colitis, including arthritis, iritis and skin lesions. Colitis arthropathy usually begins with painful swelling of a large joint, usually a knee or ankle, less commonly a joint of the upper limb. Joint symptons tend to appear when the colitis is active and rarely continue after colectomy. About 3 per cent of patients also have ankylosing spondylitis and almost 20 per cent have sacro-iliitis. Episcleritis and iritis are the commonest disorders of the eye found in ulcerative colitis. The most common cutaneous manifestations of ulcerative colitis are erythema nodosum and pyoderma gangrenosa.

## Investigations

Sigmoidoscopy is essential. The appearance of the mucosa depends upon the stage of the disease. The mucosa normally has a pale pink appearance. It becomes hyperaemic and bleeds easily. Frank ulceration is rarely seen. A biopsy should be taken and histological examination will show acute and/or chronic inflammatory changes together with crypt abscesses.

It is particularly important to identify infectious causes of colitis – especially those caused by *Entamoeba histolytica, Clostridium difficile* and *Campylobacter jejuni.* All cause sigmoidoscopic appearances similar to those in ulcerative colitis. Entamoeba may be identified on biopsy specimens or by means of the amoebic complement fixation test. Clostridium and campylobacter are both cultured from the stool; examination of which is essential in all patients with inflammatory bowel disease.

Radiological examination of the colon is contraindicated in both pregnancy and an acute exacerbation of colitis. However, if medical treatment fails, it is important to remember that patients with a long history of colitis or extensive involvement of the colon are at an increased risk of developing carcinoma of the colon.

## Treatment

In the majority of cases, corticosteroids can induce a remission during an acute attack of colitis; the milder the disease the better the response. Sulphasalazine also induces remission and reduces the risk of relapse provided it is taken continuously.

When medical treatment fails, ileostomy and proctocolectomy are curative. There are also patients whose illness is so severe that immediate surgical treatment is life saving. Peritonitis, perforation and toxic dilatation are all indications for immediate surgery and formation of a permanent ileostomy. In general, this should be undertaken in specialist centres as these have a considerably lower mortality for such procedures. If it occurs in late pregnancy there should be concurrent delivery by Caesarian section.

There is no suggestion that the fertility of women with ulcerative colitis is impaired.

Ulcerative colitis does not have an adverse effect on the progress of a pregnancy. There is no reported increase in the frequency of congenital abnormalities, spontaneous abortions or stillbirths. The management of a patient with ulcerative colitis should be the same whether pregnant or not. Neither sulphasalazine nor corticosteroids present a hazard to the developing fetus. Milk restriction can be helpful in the non-pregnant woman, but in view of its importance as a source of protein and calcium it should not be excluded from the diet of patients who are pregnant, unless they have a milk allergy.

In patients with quiescent disease at the onset of pregnancy there is an excellent chance that the ulcerative colitis will remain inactive throughout the gestation. If there is to be a recurrence, it usually occurs in the first trimester or in the puerperium and pregnancy is best avoided when the disease is active. Patients who first develop ulcerative colitis during pregnancy or the puerperium are most at risk, and usually have severe disease with a 15 per cent maternal mortality. The introduction of steroid therapy and the use of clear criteria for emergency surgical intervention, even during pregnancy, have probably reduced this figure in recent years.

McEwan (1972) reviewed a small group of five patients who underwent surgery during the antenatal period and four immediately postpartum. There was a fetal mortality of 44 per cent and a maternal mortality of 33 per cent. Although these figures probably reflect the severity of the disease, surgery should be avoided if possible, but not at risk of the mother's life.

The majority of patients with an ileostomy have successful pregnancies and deliver vaginally. Intestinal complications are unusual; but obstruction will lead to abdominal distension. Some of these patients will settle with conservative measures. Stomal complications are very common, however, and the stoma care nurse should be involved throughout the pregnancy.

**Table 8.1** Outcome of pregnancies in patients with an ileostomy for ulcerative colitis (Modifed from Fielding, 1976)

|  | Percentage of total |
| --- | --- |
| Live births | 87.5 % |
| Vaginal delivery | 75.0 % |
| Spontaneous abortion | 9.4 % |
| Therapeutic abortions | 3.0 % |
| Stomal complications | 22.0 % |

# Irritable bowel syndrome

This condition particularly effects women, usually in their third and fourth decades, but it is not uncommon in 20 year olds. It is probably uncommon for it to be newly diagnosed in pregnancy. The major complaints are of abdominal pain and a change in bowel habit. The pain may be intermittent or continuous. It is often relieved by defaecation. The majority of patients have intermittent diarrhoea, which often alternates with constipation. At this time the stool is small and pellet-like and the patient may have difficulty in defaecation. A sensation of abdominal distension, particularly related to meals is common. On examination the patient is well but may have some tenderness over the colon. Sigmoidoscopy may show spasm of the colon although this is an unreliable sign.

## Investigations

The diagnosis is really made by excluding other causes of abdominal pain and discomfort associated with a change in bowel habit. This would include a barium enema when the patient is not pregnant.

## Treatment

A simple and safe approach to this condition has been to increase the bulk of faeces by providing a high fibre diet. A similar effect is obtained by the use of bulk laxatives such as methyl cellulose and ispaghula husks. The provision of a high fibre diet will include such dietary items as wheat bran (44 g of dietary fibre/100 g of food); bran cereal (27 g), beans (25 g), wheat cereals (13 g) and muesli (7 g). Patients are advised to use products made from whole meal flour.

Recently peppermint oil capsules have been shown to relieve the colic and distension associated with irritable bowel syndrome, but they may exacerbate the heartburn of pregnancy. There are a number of antispasmodic agents and psychotropic drugs which are effective in relieving the pain of colonic spasm, but their use in pregnancy cannot be recommended.

# Pancreatitis

Pancreatitis occurs in 1 in 4000 to 12 000 pregnancies. It occurs throughout pregnancy and the puerperium, but tends to be commoner in the third trimester. It is often recurrent both within an individual pregnancy and outside it. It is usually associated with biliary disease when diagnosed in pregnancy.

The majority of patients present with nausea, vomiting and pain in the abdomen or back. The skin may be mottled, with cold extremities and a tachycardia. Shock is not unusual. About 10 per cent of patients have gastro-intestinal bleeding due to peptic ulceration. Acute pancreatitis may be associated with a pleural effusion.

## Investigations

**Table 8.2** Abnormal laboratory results in acute pancreatitis

|  | Normal values in pregnancy | Abnormality in acute pancreatitis |
|---|---|---|
| *Haematology* |  |  |
| White cell count | $5-14 \times 10^9$/litre | Polymorphonuclear leucocytosis |
| Haematocrit | 30–40 % | Raised |
| *Biochemistry* |  |  |
| Blood glucose | 3–5 mmol/litre | Transient hyperglycaemia |
| Bilirubin | 2–14 $\mu$mol/litre | Jaundice |
| Serum amylase | 0–300 i.u/litre | Elevated |
| Serum lipase | 18–285 i.u/litre | Elevated |
| Calcium | 2.15–2.35 mmol/litre | Hypocalcaemia |
| Magnesium | 2.1–3.2 mmol/litre | Hypomagnesaemia |

The interpretation of serum amylase levels is difficult because the enzyme has many origins. The elevation of pancreatic amylase seen in acute pancreatitis is transient and the level bears no relationship to the degree of pancreatic damage, and may even remain within normal limits. Abnormally elevated levels may be caused by conditions other than pancreatitis.

## Treatment

This is empirical and unsatisfactory. The two main needs are:

1. *Replacement of fluid*. Six to eight litres are frequently required and should be given as normal saline or plasma if the patient is hypotensive. Such large amounts of fluid replacement should be managed with a central venous pressure line in place. Attention must be given to calcium replacement and glucose levels.
2. *Rest of the gland*. Gastric aspiration is instituted and this reduces the passage of acid into the duodenum.

The effect of pregnancy upon the outcome of pancreatitis is uncertain but it is associated with a maternal mortality as high as 20 per cent. It has been suggested that termination should be undertaken if there is a failure to respond to conservative medical therapy.

## Further reading

Corlett, R.C. and Mishell, D.R. (1972). Pancreatitis in pregnancy. *American Journal of Obstetrics and Gynecology* **113**, 281.
De Dombal, F.T., Burton, I.L. and Goligher, J.C. (1972). Crohn's disease and pregnancy. *British Medical Journal* **3**, 550.
Fielding, J.F. (1976). Inflammatory bowel disease and pregnancy.

*British Journal of Hospital Medicine* **15**, 345.

Janerot, G. and Into-Malmberg, M.B. (1979). Sulphasalazine treatment during breast feeding. *Scandinavian Journal of Gastroenterology* **14**, 869.

Martimbeau, P.W., Welch, J.S. and Weiland, L.H. (1975). Crohn's disease and pregnancy. *American Journal of Obstetrics and Gynecology* **122**, 746.

Miller, J.P. (1977). Diseases of the liver and alimentary tract. *Clinics in Obstetrics and Gynecology* **4**, 297.

Mogadam, M., Dobbins, W.O., Korelitz, B.I. and Ahmed, S.W. (1981). Pregnancy in inflammatory bowel disease: effect of sulphasalazine and corticosteroids on fetal outcome. *Gastroenterology* **80**, 72.

Norton, R.A. and Patterson, J.F. (1972). Pregnancy and regional enteritis. *Obstetrics and Gynecology* **40**, 711.

Ogborn, A.D.R. (1975). Pregnancy in patients with coeliac disease. *British Journal of Obstetrics and Gynecology* **82**, 293.

Willoughby, C.P. and Truelove, S.C. (1980). Ulcerative colitis and pregnancy. *Gut* **21**, 469.

# 9

# The acute abdomen

Pregnancy often confounds and delays the diagnosis and treatment of acute abdominal pain. This is due to a combination of the altered clinical presentation of intercurrent disease, complications of the pregnancy itself and a reluctance to perform a laparotomy. Such an attitude towards laparotomy is on the whole unjustified.

Diagnosis of an acute abdomen always requires a careful history and clinical examination as radiological examination may have to be restricted. However, with modern equipment X-ray dosages are safe for most procedures. Direct complications of the pregnancy should be excluded first and this will narrow the differential diagnosis.

## In the abdomen or in the abdominal wall?

It is a common fault to overlook the possibility of injuries to the abdominal wall. 'Pulled muscles' are quite common as the pregnant mother learns to use alternative muscle groups to achieve familiar actions. Coughing may lead to the rupture of branches of the inferior epigastric artery. On examination there are often unilateral signs and occasionally a raised tender lump in the affected muscle may be felt. There may also be an apparent rebound tenderness which is still present when the recti are made to contract by asking the patient to straight leg raise or sit up.

Treatment is expectant though some symptomatic relief can be achieved by local 'rubs' and simple analgesia may help: The injection of local anaesthetic with or without an anti-inflammatory steroid preparation is best reserved for non-pregnant women.

## Direct complications of the pregnancy
### Ectopic gestation

Mortality from this condition remains relatively high at 1 in 500 cases in the United Kingdom. Death is due to intraperitoneal haemorrhage,

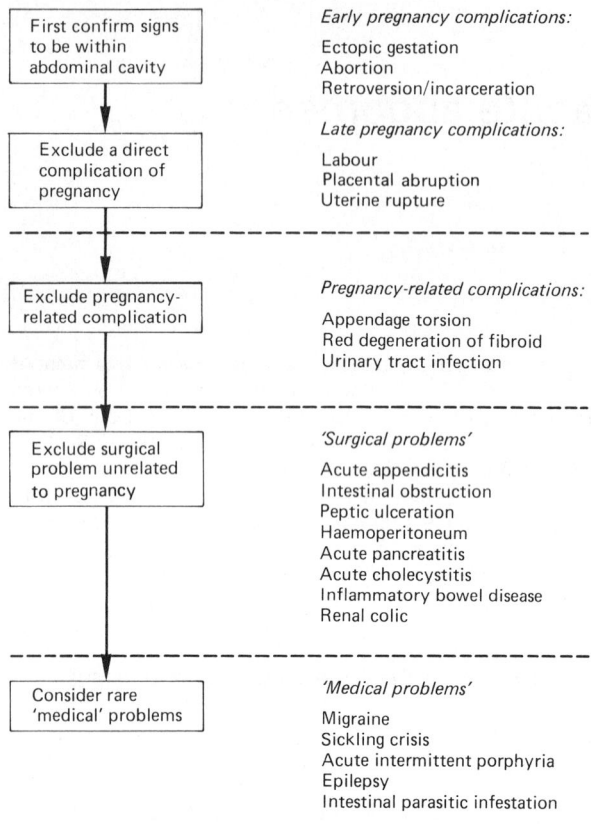

First confirm signs
to be within
abdominal cavity

*Early pregnancy complications:*

Ectopic gestation
Abortion
Retroversion/incarceration

Exclude a direct
complication of
pregnancy

*Late pregnancy complications:*

Labour
Placental abruption
Uterine rupture

Exclude pregnancy-
related complication

*Pregnancy-related complications:*

Appendage torsion
Red degeneration of fibroid
Urinary tract infection

Exclude surgical
problem unrelated
to pregnancy

*'Surgical problems'*

Acute appendicitis
Intestinal obstruction
Peptic ulceration
Haemoperitoneum
Acute pancreatitis
Acute cholecystitis
Inflammatory bowel disease
Renal colic

Consider rare
'medical' problems

*'Medical problems'*

Migraine
Sickling crisis
Acute intermittent porphyria
Epilepsy
Intestinal parasitic infestation

**Fig. 9.1**   Diagnosis of acute abdomen in pregnancy.

although other common, but seldom fatal complications include tubal abortion and tubal mole. The clinical picture is variable but careful questioning usually reveals a period of amenorrhoea or a 'light' last menstrual period. There is usually an element of vaginal bleeding but abdominal pain, fainting and shoulder pain are not necessarily present.

General examination may reveal profound shock with an obvious haemoperitoneum. Less dramatic signs include a mild pyrexia of less than 38°C and localized rebound tenderness. Pelvic findings include cervical tenderness, a 'fullness' in one fornix or a pelvic haematocoele.

Although the history and examination are rarely classical a diagnosis can usually be made. More chronic presentations can be mistaken for pelvic inflammatory disease and laparoscopy may be needed to confirm the diagnosis. Although surgical techniques are not the subject of this book it is important to emphasize the absolute necessity of an urgent laparotomy in the shocked patient with a haemoperitoneum. Any delay is likely to result in the death of the patient. Junior anaesthetists may be reluctant to take such a patient to theatre without some attempt at resuscitation but in such circumstances the location and ligation of the offending vessels is the most important initial step in successful resuscitation.

## Abortion

All forms of abortion are associated with vaginal bleeding and can present as an acute abdomen. Although septic abortion is seen less frequently today, it is often concealed by the patient, especially when it is secondary to a criminal perforation of the uterus. If peritonitis is present, intravenous antibiotic therapy as well as a laparotomy will be required.

## Retroverted gravid uterus

Patients who present with this problem are usually 11–16 weeks pregnant. Retention of urine may be the first symptom and later complications include pain and vaginal bleeding due to incarceration of the gravid uterus in the bony pelvis. If incarceration were uncorrected, gangrene, septicaemia and death would be potential sequelae.

Catheterization and adoption of a prone position by the patient for 24–72 hours usually results in spontaneous anteversion of the uterus. Digital displacement and subsequent insertion of a Hodge pessary may be necessary if this fails. The pessary will maintain anteversion until the uterus is larger than the bony pelvis and the danger has passed.

## Placental abruption

In late pregnancy, placental abruption, especially of the concealed variety, is often associated with acute abdominal pain and shock. The signs may be confused with such upper abdominal problems as a perforated peptic ulcer.

Examination of the abdomen reveals a tense 'woody' uterine wall with a uterus which is big-for-dates due to internal haemorrhage. On auscultation fetal heart sounds may not be heard. Labour usually supervenes.

## Labour

It is common for young girls who have concealed or 'denied' their pregnancy to present at a hospital casualty department with colicky abdominal pain. Examination usually confirms the diagnosis, but in a very tense individual who refuses a vaginal examination and has excessive abdominal guarding, the presence of a fetal heart beat may be the only absolute confirmation of the diagnosis. Sometimes it is difficult to convince such individuals of their pregnant state even as late as the second stage of labour!

## Uterine rupture

Rupture is usually associated with previous uterine surgery. It may occur acutely during labour with searing abdominal pain and the signs of a haemoperitoneum, or in a silent form which is discovered when the patient reports cessation of fetal movements.

# Pregnancy related problems

## Urinary tract infection

As mentioned in Chapter 5 infection of the urinary tract is common in pregnancy. When the upper tract is affected, the presentation may be that of an acute abdomen. A helpful history of frequency, dysuria and loin pain may be present and nausea and vomiting are particularly common.

Examination can reveal tenderness even to the extent of apparent peritonism over the course of the ureters. If this occurs, however, there is almost always tenderness in one or both renal angles.

Immediate microscopy of the urine should confirm the diagnosis by showing significant numbers of leucocytes and erythrocytes. Treatment is by intravenous antibiotics and analgesics.

## Torsion of ovarian cyst/uterine appendage

The uterine appendages undergo considerable reorientation during pregnancy and the puerperium. Rotation and torsion of a normal appendage is rare but this is not so if the appendage carries a cystic ovary. Most ovarian cysts in this age group are dermoids which are heavy and have long pedicles which predispose them to torsion. The majority of cases occur during pregnancy but the puerperium is also a time of risk owing to rapid involution of the uterus.

The clinical picture is of intermittent colicky abdominal pain which increases in frequency and intensity as the ischaemic damage progresses. Vomiting is common. Examination may reveal a tender cystic mass and pyrexia. Ultrasound can be of help, but in the absence of calcified structures such as teeth, dermoid cysts and haemorrhagic cysts tend to look like fibroids. Only in the presence of known fibroids can a laparotomy be delayed.

### Red degeneration of a uterine fibroid

Fibroids may grow rapidly in pregnancy due to oestrogens and increased vascularity. Arterial thrombosis and venous engorgement together result in red degeneration. The patient is pyrexial and has a tender mass which mimics ovarian cyst torsion or appendicitis. A prior knowledge of the presence of fibroids is invaluable.

When examination reveals such a tender mass with evidence of peritonism, laparotomy is often necessary to exclude a life threatening condition. Only incarcerated fibroids or those on long slim pedicles need to be removed in pregnancy. In other situations the risk of haemorrhage is unacceptable during pregnancy.

## Miscellaneous pregnancy related complications

In particularly severe cases, or in patients whose pain threshold is low, pelvic arthropathy of pregnancy can present with low abdominal pain which is exacerbated by walking. Separation of the symphysis pubis is easily demonstrated in the standing position, when the patient changes weight bearing from one leg to the other.

Many such pains go undiagnosed but syndromes that have been described include 'round ligament strain' and the recently described twelfth rib syndrome. Round ligament strain is a doubtful entity though the location of the pain is often convincing. Twelfth rib syndrome is an intercostal neuralgia which causes pain in the loin and upper abdominal quadrant.

## Problems unrelated to pregnancy

### Acute appendicitis

Acute appendicitis complicates 1 in 4000 pregnancies and is attended by more problems than in non-pregnant women. This is almost certainly because of delayed intervention.

In early pregnancy, the clinical picture is often identical to that in the non-pregnant patient with central, colicky abdominal pain which localizes to the right iliac fossa. The pain can be accompanied by some vomiting and loose bowel motions. In later pregnancy the caecum and appendix are displaced upwards and laterally. Pain is often maximal at the waistline and in the flank. If the uterus is interposed between the examining hand and the appendix, guarding may not occur. Likewise rectal examination can be unhelpful because the appendix and inflamed peritoneum are pushed up into the abdomen out of reach of the examining finger.

The condition is most frequently confused with acute urinary tract infection, though in the latter case loin tenderness and pyrexia should be discriminating factors. Investigations are usually unhelpful and the diagnosis is confirmed at laparotomy.

## Paralytic ileus

Paralytic ileus is rarely seen in pregnancy but it may occur in association with a haemoperitoneum or abdominal sepsis. A true pregnancy ileus has been described and occurs after delivery.

Ileus is characterized by symptoms which include vomiting, abdominal pain and distension. Marked dilatation of the colon may occur in isolation, so that bowel sounds may still be present on ausculation.

Diagnosis is by abdominal plain X-ray. Conventional treatment by nasogastric aspiration and intravenous electrolytes is indicated. Occasionally, however, a caecostomy or colostomy may be the only way to relieve colonic dilatation.

## Intestinal obstruction

This is uncommon unless predisposing factors such as adhesions are present. Carcinoma of the rectum or colon although uncommon can present in this age group. Symptoms are similar to those in the non-pregnant state with colicky abdominal pain as the predominant feature. Vomiting is a late complication.

Examination reveals distension in the area above the uterus and hyperactive bowel sounds on auscultation. The diagnosis may be confirmed by abdominal plain X-ray. Conservative treatment with nasogastric suction and intravenous fluid replacement should normally be tried before resorting to laparotomy.

## Cholecystitis

Cholecystitis is perhaps seen more often in the reproductive age group than formerly. In pregnancy it typically presents with colicky pain in the right upper quadrant. There may be a pyrexia and some degree of jaundice. Maximum tenderness occurs over the region of the gall bladder itself.

Management of the first attack should be conservative with nasogastric aspiration, intravenous fluids, analgesics, antispasmodics and perhaps antibiotics. Radiological and surgical intervention should be left until the puerperium. Biliary surgery in pregnancy is often technically difficult but may sometimes be necessary.

## Renal calculi

Renal colic rarely occurs for the first time in pregnancy but when it does the classic 'loin to groin' pain is usually present and examination reveals poorly localized tenderness in the relevant flank. Loin tenderness is only likely if a significant hydronephrosis has developed. Accompanying signs of urinary tract infection may also be present.

The diagnosis is by ultrasound or modified intravenous urography if there is some clinical doubt. Treatment is conservative with analgesics and antispasmodics. However, if there is a total failure to control symptoms or there is evidence of impending renal damage, surgery is indicated and this may be by an endoscopic or open approach.

## Haemoperitoneum

Ruptured ectopic pregnancy apart, the occurrence of a haemoperitoneum is rare. Blunt trauma as in road traffic accidents can cause haemorrhage particularly from the liver or spleen. Spontaneous rupture of the spleen or utero-ovarian veins may occur and the possibility of uterine rupture should be remembered.

Clinical signs are variable but often include hypovolaemic shock and abdominal distension. A degree of peritonism is likely as is dullness in the flanks. Paralytic ileus may supervene.

Laparotomy is indicated and where the source of haemorrhage is in doubt a multidisciplinary surgical team is necessary.

# Medical causes of acute abdominal pain

A number of medical conditions, such as diabetes, may cause acute abdominal pain. The most important of these is acute intermittent porphyria which is sometimes first diagnosed during the pregnancy. Other possibilities include sickling crisis, migraine, epilepsy and intestinal infestation. Medical causes of abdominal pain are rare and should usually enter the differential diagnosis at a relatively late stage.

# Radiological investigations during pregnancy

There has long been debate about the effects on the fetus of diagnostic X-rays. Reports of increased rates of congenital abnormalities and increased childhood cancer exist but are open to differing statistical interpretations.

Modern plain abdominal X-rays deliver dosages to the fetus within the millirad range and are not realistically dangerous. Investigations using contrast media tend to cause greater exposure and are generally best avoided. If, however, the mother's health is severely threatened then she should not be denied a potentially helpful diagnostic procedure.

# Laparotomy in pregnancy

Fear of precipitating a preterm labour often leads to a postponement of a laparotomy. Such a delay is frequently to the detriment of both mother and baby and is usually unjustified. It is not the laparotomy but the underlying condition which may stimulate uterine activity or contribute to fetal compromise. Thus the pyrexia and inflammatory processes of acute appendicitis are the main cause of early labour.

Where the risk of preterm labour has been identified, use of a tocolytic agent such as ritodrine or a narcotic analgaesic is helpful. Any attempt at the suppression of preterm labour must however be in the absence of fetal compromise as shown by the presence of a satisfactory fetal heart rate pattern. Surgery of this nature is therefore best performed close to a suitably equipped neonatal unit.

# 10

# Pregnancy and liver disease

It is unusual for a patient with chronic liver disease to become pregnant, but in most cases no alteration in management is required. Some liver function tests are effected by pregnancy but the histology of liver biopsies taken from normal pregnant patients show only minor non-specific changes which include an increase in nuclear size and in the frequency of binucleate cells. Occasionally there is a mild lymphocytic infiltration of the portal areas.

**Table 10.1** Changes in liver function tests during pregnancy

| Test | Effect of pregnancy |
|---|---|
| 1.  Alkaline phosphatase | The level is increased from 5th week to term |
| 2.  Total cholesterol | This is raised throughout pregnancy |
| 3.  Total protein | During the first trimester the level falls to 85 % of the non-pregnant value and remains at this level during the remainder of the pregnancy |
|       i.  Albumin | The level falls to 66 % of the non-pregnant value by term |
|      ii.  Globulin | $\alpha$ and $\beta$ fractions increase, while $\gamma$ globulins show a small fall |
| 4.  Bromsulphthalein dye test (BSP). Seldom performed today | In the standard test 5 mg/kg are given and a blood sample is taken at 45 minutes. During pregnancy there is an increase in uptake of BSP from plasma, a two fold increase in the return of dye to plasma and a reduction by half to two-thirds in the elimination of dye into the bile and an alteration in the proportion of dye lost from liver cells through plasma and bile respectively. The overall effect may lead to dye retention at 45 minutes up to five times non-pregnant values. BSP does not cross the placenta |

# Liver disease peculiar to pregnancy

## Intrahepatic cholestasis of pregnancy

*Synonyms*
Hepatosis of pregnancy, benign recurrent cholestasis of pregnancy, idiopathic jaundice of pregnancy and pruritus gravidarum.

This condition may effect as many as 1 in a 1000 pregnancies and is characterized by increasingly severe pruritus which usually begins in the third trimester of pregnancy. Some cases progress to clinical jaundice, with typical features of cholestasis including pale stools and dark urine. In contrast to patients with infectious hepatitis who have a similar presentation, the patient usually feels well. Jaundice and pruritus remit rapidly following delivery.

### Investigations

Serum bilirubin increases to 103 to 171 $\mu$mol/litre and remains constant until delivery. Most of it is direct-reacting bilirubin. Alkaline phosphatase and 5$'$ nucleotidase levels are moderately increased, whereas $\gamma$ Guanosine triphosphate (GTP) characteristically remains normal. Aminotransferases are also elevated. Bile acids are raised and are considered to be responsible for the pruritus. Bromsulphthalein (BSP) dye retention is prolonged due to a reduction in transport maxima. It may remain abnormal for some months after pregnancy in contrast to other liver function tests which quickly return to normal.

Liver biopsy reveals centrilobular cholestasis with rather delicate bile thrombi and minimal inflammation in the portal tracts. Although an association with gall stones has been described this seldom leads to duct obstruction and ultrasound will distinguish the two conditions.

### Management

Recently, an increased incidence of premature labour has been noticed in patients with intrahepatic cholestasis of pregnancy. The effect on the fetus is probably minimal although it is possible that there is an increased occurrence of fetal death and postpartum haemorrhage. Treatment may be required for symptomatic relief of pruritus, and cholestyramine in doses of 4 g, orally, four times a day, is of value. If the drug is used for a lengthy period, vitamin A and D, and water soluble vitamin K supplements should be given. After delivery, vitamin K should be given prophylactically to mother and child to prevent bleeding. Special care facilities may be needed because of the increased incidence of prematurity.

The contraceptive pill has been associated with cholestatic jaundice. There is a selective interference of oestrogens with the hepatic excretion of bilirubin and this usually appears within the first six cycles of oral contraception. Women who develop this condition appear to be at risk of intrahepatic cholestasis of pregnancy, which in itself may be a precursor of primary biliary cirrhosis.

## Acute fatty liver of pregnancy

*Synonyms*

Pernicious steatosis, acute fatty metamorphosis of pregnancy and obstetrical acute yellow atrophy.

This syndrome is a rare cause of jaundice which mainly affects obese primigravid women in the last trimester and even at birth. There is a dramatic onset of abdominal pain, vomiting, severe headache, tachycardia and jaundice. The patient may become oliguric, increasingly drowsy and start to bleed from the gastro-intestinal tract. Muscle pain and renal failure are frequent.

About 50 cases have been reported with a maternal mortality of greater than 80 per cent and a fetal loss in 70 per cent of cases. In cases where the mother survived, the fetal loss was reduced to only 40 per cent. Death may occur up to several days after delivery, but if the mother survives her ultimate prognosis is good. A similar disease, has occurred after the intravenous administration of large doses of old tetracycline for pyelonephritis in pregnant women.

### Investigations

Serum bilirubin is only mildly elevated and rarely reaches 171 $\mu$ mol/litre. Aminotransferase and alkaline phosphatase activities are only mildly increased, uric acid and blood urea are usually high and hypoglycaemia is common and difficult to correct. Blood coagulation is severely impaired.

Histology of the liver typically shows panlobular fatty change with periportal sparing and the absence of hepatocellular necrosis or significant inflammatory infiltrate, distinguishes the condition from fulminant viral hepatitis.

### Management

Treatment is symptomatic for hepatic and renal failure. This will require:

1. Intensive care monitoring. Cardiac arrhythmias may occur in up to a third of patients.
2. Intravenous fluid therapy. Special attention to hypoglycaemia must be given and adequate 10 per cent dextrose provided. Additional intravenous glucose is given as required. 600 mmol of potassium may be required daily to maintain a normal plasma potassium level.
3. Correction of bleeding diathesis. As vitamin K has little effect on the low prothrombin index, at least 3 units of fresh frozen

plasma or cryoprecipitate are needed daily.
4. Alleviation of encephalopathy. The protein load in the gastro-intestinal tract is reduced by increasing intestinal transit by the use of laxatives to rid the gut of accumulated blood or protein. The intake of protein by mouth should be reduced below 20 g/24 hour. Lactulose is of particular value in the presence of concomitant renal failure, as it increases stool frequency, and probably results in a decreased ammonia production. Ammonia may be involved in the aetiology of hepatic encephalopathy.

If the infant survives, it does not appear to be affected and the maternal liver recovers completely in the small number of survivors. Further pregnancies are possible and safe.

## Spontaneous rupture of the liver

About 50 cases of spontaneous rupture of the liver associated with pregnancy have been reported since 1844. Rupture usually occurs in the last trimester of multiparous women. There is sudden onset of epigastric or right upper quadrant pain, nausea and vomiting. This may be associated with hypotension, shock and abdominal swelling.

### Investigations

The sudden deterioration usually precludes any investigation other than paracentesis which reveals fresh blood. In cases with a small haemorrhagic ooze radionucleïde scanning, ultrasound or hepatic angiography have helped in the diagnosis. Liver function tests may show a hepatitic pattern and be associated with disseminated intravascular coagulation.

### Treatment

During surgical repair of the tear which may be by oversewing, packing, hepatic artery ligation or partial hepatectomy, the fetus should be delivered by Caesarian section. Despite treatment, maternal mortality is high and may be due to rebleeding, hepatic and renal failure, right lower lobe collapse and the formation of subdiaphragmatic abscesses.

If the rupture is antenatal only 14 per cent of fetuses survive.

## Intercurrent liver disease occurring during pregnancy

Viral hepatitis is probably the commonest cause of jaundice during pregnancy.

# Hepatitis A

*Synonyms*

Infectious hepatitis, short incubation hepatitis and MS-1 hepatitis. The prodromal symptoms vary in severity and duration, and patients may present with jaundice. The appearance of jaundice is usually associated with an improvement in anorexia, nausea and lassitude. There is tenderness in the right upper quadrant and the liver is usually enlarged. The urine is dark and stools are pale.

European and American studies have shown that pregnancy does not worsen the effect of hepatitis A. In such parts of the world as India however, it is the third commonest cause of maternal mortality and may be associated with an increased fetal mortality.

### Investigations

Hepatitis A antigen and antibody can be detected in stools or serum by immune electron microscopy. Unfortunately this is time consuming and its value is limited. Complement fixation and immune aherence haemagglutination techniques have been developed for the detection of antibody in serum and antigen and antibody may be detected by radio-immunoassay. Hepatitis A virus appears in the prodromal stage and is associated with a transient viraemia. It is undetectable in stool or serum once jaundice has appeared.

Confirmation of hepatitis A remains difficult and the most important investigation in any case of viral hepatitis is exclusion of an infection by hepatitis B. In most clinical laboratories the identification of B antigen is the only readily available way of distinguishing between hepatitis A and B.

### Treatment

During the acute attack patients may be anorexic and nauseated. Bed-rest and restriction of fatty food may be of help. The patient should receive adequate hydration, if necessary, by an intravenous route. Because of the possibility of premature delivery and fetal death, women should receive prophylactic immunization with 0.02 ml immune serum globulin/kg of body weight given intramuscularly, even when they are only casual contacts of patients with hepatitis A. Passive immunization is effective in protecting 80-90 per cent of contacts for up to 6 months, if administered within 2 weeks of exposure.

# Hepatitis B

*Synonyms*

Serum hepatitis, long-incubation hepatitis, MS-2 hepatitis, hepatitis B surface antigen (HBs Ag)-positive, Hepatitis-associated antigen

(HAA) positive hepatitis and Australia antigen-positive hepatitis. Although this infection is common in drug addicts, other people are at risk and the symptoms are similar to those of hepatitis A infections.

A proportion of patients develop chronic liver disease, some have persistent hepatitis, whilst others become carriers of hepatitis B. The majority recover and very few die of the acute disease.

The course of hepatitis B infection does not appear to be altered by pregnancy, although this may not be true in developing countries. Most studies have shown an increased frequency of premature birth, but the suggestions that there was a greater frequency of congenital malformations and Down's syndrome have not been confirmed.

## Investigations

A number of techniques are available for detection of hepatitis B infection. However, the detection of 'e' antigen and 'e' antibody are of particular importance in pregnancy; and this may be done by passive haemagglutination or radio-immunoassay. The presence of 'e' antibody is associated with low infectivity, including transmission to the fetus.

The condition must be distinguished from fatty liver of pregnancy and cholestasis. Liver function tests and a screen for Australian antigen must be performed.

## Treatment

Patients should be given passive immunization and vaccination should be considered. Vaccination is not effective for 6 months and so those at risk should have passive immunization as well as vaccination.

If the mother has intractable nausea and vomiting during the pregnancy she will require hospital admission to maintain fluid and carbohydrate intake. Because liver glycogen stores are impaired, hypoglycaemia may develop. If the patient develops hepatic failure with ascites, peripheral oedema and encephalopathy, the prognosis is grave.

About two thirds of children born to mothers with acute hepatitis B late in pregnancy or during the postpartum period will develop evidence of infection within 1–6 months. How many of these children will develop chronic liver disease or hepatoma is unknown, but because of the risk, high titre anti-B immune globulins should be administered soon after birth and the injection repeated at monthly intervals for 6 months. The place of vaccination with inactivated hepatitis B is the subject of current research.

The risk to staff and other patients from an infected mother is best met by isolating mother and child, use of double gloves and careful handling of infected material.

## Budd-Chiari syndrome

*Synonym*
Hepatic venous outflow obstruction
Patients develop a painful, tender liver with ascites. Subsequently, portal hypertension and oesophageal varices appear. Most of the cases develop postpartum and the fetus is not at risk. When it does occur in pregnancy intra-uterine death is inevitable.

### Investigations

In the postpartum patient, liver scanning with $^{99}Te^m$ sulphur colloid is a useful screening test. Characteristically, the antero-posterior scan shows central uptake of radio colloid in the caudate lobe with a reduced uptake in the right lobe. Catheterization may reveal obstruction of the hepatic veins or the inferior vena cava. A liver biopsy shows thrombosis in the central veins and sinusoids with interlobular congestion.

### Treatment

The outcome of portosystemic shunting is unimpressive and the prognosis is very poor. Up to 50 per cent of the patients die in the postoperative period.

## Gall-stones

There is an impression that biliary disease is relatively common in pregnant women; although biliary tree obstruction is rare. In pregnancy there is a reduction in the rate of excretion of chenodeoxycholic acid and in the rate of gall bladder emptying which both lead to stone formation.

### Investigation

Plain X-ray of the abdomen is unlikely to demonstrate a radio-lucent stone and cholangiography is of no value in jaundice. Ultrasound examination is the technique of choice.

### Treatment

This is unaltered by pregnancy and surgery should be undertaken in cases with common bile duct obstruction. However, when available, endoscopic removal of the stones should be considered.

# Pregnancy and pre-existing liver disease

## Gilbert's syndrome

Synonym
Unconjugated hyperbilirubinaemia.

Between 3 and 7 per cent of the population show an elevated level of unconjugated bilirubin in the plasma, which is often detected by incidental laboratory examination. An increase in the level of bilirubin may be caused by fasting, pregnancy or following surgery, but patients are mainly asymptomatic.

### Investigations

Liver biopsy is helpful but seldom necessary. It is important to exclude haemolysis and acquired liver disease.

### Treatment

Although unconjugated bilirubin crosses the placenta and will cause kernicterus, there have been no studies of pregnancy in this common disease. Its effect on the fetus is unknown, but careful observation of bilirubin levels will be needed during the neonatal period.

## Dubin–Johnson syndrome

*Synonym*
Conjugated hyperbilirubinaemia.
This is an autosomal recessive disease in which there is impaired excretion of bile which leads to jaundice and occasionally hepatosplenomegaly. In pregnancy the jaundice deepens and may result in abortion or stillbirth.

### Investigations

The liver function tests in this condition are usually normal although a liver biopsy shows melanin pigment granules in the centrilobular areas.

### Treatment

No active treatment of this disease is required during pregnancy. Conjugated bilirubin does not collect in nervous tissue and there is no risk of kernicterus developing in the fetus.

# Wilson's disease

*Synonym*
Hepatolenticular degeneration.
This condition is rare and due to a defect in copper metabolism. The accumulation of toxic amounts of copper begins in infancy, but the deposits are limited for years to the liver. Patients develop fatigue, jaundice, portal hypertension with its clinical manifestations of oedema, ascites and splenomegaly, the neuropsychiatric changes of tremor, fluctuating rigidity and a deterioration in personality. Primary or secondary amenorrhoea is common in women.

### Investigations

In early stages where copper accumulates in the liver, neurological signs and the rusty brown Kayser–Fleischer ring at the periphery of the cornea are absent. The liver function tests are normal, but serum caeruloplasmin concentrations are raised even after extensive 'decoppering'. A liver biopsy may show fibrosis or even a picture similar to chronic active hepatitis. A definitive diagnosis may be made by estimating the copper concentration in dry liver. It is usually between 0.3–0.8 $\mu$mol/g in healthy individuals, but may range from 4–47 $\mu$mol/g in untreated patients with Wilson's disease.

### Treatment

Penicillamine in daily doses of 1–2 g, increases the urinary excretion of copper and therefore reduces the concentration of the metal in the body. Patients with untreated Wilson's disease are subfertile and high uterine copper concentrations may be responsible for an increased incidence of spontaneous abortions. Treatment with penicillamine appears to correct infertility and lead to successful completion of pregnancy, especially in those patients with mainly neurological rather than hepatic symptoms. Penicillamine does not appear to affect the fetus and should be continued throughout the pregnancy, but as it depletes maternal stores of pyridoxine this should be given as a supplement. If a Caesarian section is planned then penicillamine should be withheld temporarily as it may impair wound healing.

# Chronic active hepatitis

This is a progressive destruction of the liver with a prolonged course. Characteristically the disease affects young women. The majority of the patients have hepatomegaly and many have splenomegaly.

### Investigations

The disease is associated with the presence of antinuclear factor (ANF) in the serum. The patient may be jaundiced with a bilirubin of between 50–170 $\mu$mol/litre and serum transaminase levels are moderately elevated. A liver biopsy shows characteristic changes of an inflammatory infiltrate in portal tracts and fibroblastic destruction of the liver parenchyma. This results in isolation of liver cells at the interface between parenchyma and collagen and has been called piecemeal necrosis.

### Treatment

The mortality from this condition is high and in untreated series 50 per cent of patients are dead within 5 years. Prednisone alone (20 mg) or in combination (10 mg) with 50 mg azathioprine significantly improves life expectancy with histological resolution and the return of biochemistry to normal.

The fertility of patients with chronic active hepatitis is reduced, but this particularly responds to treatment. Pregnancy does not appear to alter the course of the disease, although most fetuses are born early and are of low birth-weight. Treatment with corticosteroids should certainly be continued throughout the pregnancy, but it is probably desirable to withdraw azathioprine. However, the use of steroids suppresses fetal oestriol and prevents its use as an index of placental function.

## Primary biliary cirrhosis

This disease particularly effects middle aged women. The onset is often insidious and starts as pruritus often during pregnancy. The pruritus may persists after delivery, although it can remit only to reappear years later. Jaundice usually appears some months after the onset of itching and is of the cholestatic type with darkening of urine and pale stools. Both liver and spleen are usually enlarged and associated with oesophageal varices.

### Investigations

Initially serum bilirubin is low. Serum alkaline phosphatase is raised and an elevated 5' nucleotidase confirms its biliary origin. Almost all patients with primary biliary cirrhosis have antimitochondrial antibody in their serum; but it is also to be found in about 20 per cent of patients with chronic active hepatitis and occasionally in thyroiditis and gastritis.

A liver biopsy shows progressive granulomatous injury and finally loss of intrahepatic bile ducts.

**Treatment**

The course of the disease is unpredictable. Nowadays many cases are diagnosed by the demonstration of antimitochondrial antibody in the serum of non-jaundiced patients. However, once jaundice has developed the average life expectancy is 5 years. Calorie and protein intake must be maintained; although fat should be restricted to 40 g in the jaundiced patient. If the thrombin time is prolonged regular vitamin K (10 mg daily by the intramuscular route) is necessary. Although the pruritus may be controlled by cholestyramine this drug must be used with caution during pregnancy. Bone thinning and fractures may be a problem and patients will benefit from sunlight, 100 000 units of vitamin D intramuscularly once a month and up to 900 mg of microcrystalline hydroxyapatite compound (MCHC) daily. Steroids, azathioprine and penicillamine seem to offer little benefit to the patient.

Although patients are now diagnosed earlier, pregnancy is unusual and this is still probably related to age. In most reports less than half of pregnancies have successfully reached term, and maternal death can occur.

# Further reading

Lockhart, D., Katz, S.S., Lisbona, R. and Mishkin, S. (1981). Oral contraceptives and liver disease. *Canadian Medical Association Journal* **124**, 993.

Steven, M.M. (1981). Pregnancy and liver disease. *Gut* **22**, 592.

Wands, J.R. (1979). Viral hepatitis and its effect on pregnancy. *Clinical Obstetrics and Gynecology* **22**, 301.

Wright, R., Alberti, K.G.M.M., Karran, S. and Millward-Sadler, G.H. (1979). *Liver and Biliary Disease*. W.B. Saunders.

Walshe, J.M. (1977). Pregnancy in Wilson's disease. *Quarterly Journal of Medicine* **46**, 73.

# 11

# Haematological disorders

One of the commonest problems in antenatal care is a progressive fall in haemoglobin, particularly during the last trimester. Causes range from a simple physiological increase in plasma volume to serious underlying haematological disorders. Any definition of anaemia must be arbitrary and the World Health Organisation (WHO) have suggested 11.0 g/dl as the level below which anaemia exists in pregnant women. Anaemia may be the result of nutritional deficiency, haemolysis, a hypoplastic marrow or a neoplastic process such as lymphoma or leukaemia.

## Blood volume changes in pregnancy

During pregnancy the plasma volume increases by about 1 litre, or 1500 ml in the case of a twin pregnancy. The red cell mass increases by about 300 ml and this results in a relative haemodilution with a fall in the haematocrit from 41 per cent to 35 per cent and a parallel fall in the haemoglobin concentration to as low as 10 g/dl. These changes start

**Table 11.1** Haematological values during pregnancy

|  | Pregnancy 12 weeks | 24 weeks | 36 weeks | Non-pregnant values |
|---|---|---|---|---|
| White cell count ($\times 10^9$/litre) | 5–12 | 6–15 | 6–14 | 4–11 |
| Red cell count ($\times 10^{12}$/litre) | 3.5–4.6 | 3.3–4.3 | 3.4–4.4 | 3.8–5.8 |
| Haemoglobin (g/dl) | 10.8–13.2 | 10.5–12.9 | 10.6–13.8 | 11.5–16.5 |
| Haematocrit (%) | 31–39 | 30–38 | 32–40 | 41.5–42.5 |
| Mean cell volume (fl) | 80–94 | 84–98 | 84–98 | 77–93 |
| Mean cell haemoglobin (pg) | 27.5–31.5 | 28.5–32.5 | 28.5–32.5 | 27–32 |
| Mean cell haemoglobin concentration (g/dl) | 32–36 | 32–36 | 32–36 | 31–35 |
| Serum ferritin (micrograms/litre) | 30 | 10 | 6 | 9–120 |

early in pregnancy but are most marked towards the end of the second trimester, and the lowest haemoglobin concentration is recorded at about 34 weeks.

The increase in erythropoiesis is dependent on normal marrow function. Mild infection, such as a urinary infection, or a previously compensated anaemia such as $\beta$-thalassaemia minor are potent causes of anaemia during the late stages of pregnancy or the puerperium. These anaemias resolve in the weeks following delivery.

## *Nutritional anaemias*

## Iron deficiency anaemia

In a classic study of healthy young college women of good socio-economic status two-thirds had an absence or deficiency of their iron stores (Scott and Pritchard, 1967). Consequently many women enter pregnancy without adequate iron stores and in a study of pregnant patients living in British industrial cities 10–31 per cent had haemoglobin levels below 10 g/dl (Scott, 1962). During pregnancy a mother loses 250–400 mg of iron to the fetus, particularly during the last trimester. The placenta also contains about 150 mg of iron which is lost to the mother at parturition. If a woman is to remain in iron balance she will need to absorb about 2 mg of iron each day above her normal daily requirement of 1.5 mg.

Lassitude, weakness, fatigue, dyspnoea on exertion and palpitations are common symptoms. Changes can occur in the nails leading to longitudinal ridging and in severe cases they become concave or spoon shaped (koilonychia). Atrophy of the papillae of the tongue results in atrophic glossitis. Augular stomatitis with redness, soreness and cracking at the angles of the mouth may occur.

Fetal consequences of maternal iron deficiency are negligible. Even in the face of marked maternal iron deficiency the fetus will take iron from the mother. The association of prematurity and anaemia certainly exists, but it is less clear that there is a direct association with iron deficiency.

### Investigation

The anaemia of iron deficiency is characteristically a hypochromic microcytic anaemia. However, in the early stages hypochromia may be present without definite microcytosis. The blood film may show hypochromia, anisocytosis and poikilocytosis. Variation in shape is usual and elliptical forms are common. Target cells are often present. However, all these changes are less obvious than they are in the non-pregnant woman.

The mean corpuscular haemoglobin (MCH) and mean cell volume (MCV) are lowered in the presence of iron deficiency anaemia, rather than physiological dilution. In true iron deficiency the total iron binding capacity (TIBC) is increased over 98.5 $\mu$mol/litre and the serum iron may be below 9 $\mu$mol/litre. Serum ferritin is also low, but these last three measurements are only necessary if there is no response to oral iron therapy and parenteral treatment is being considered. The most conclusive diagnostic feature of iron deficiency is the absence of stainable iron in marrow fragments obtained by marrow aspiration, although this is seldom necessary for diagnosis.

## Treatment

### Oral administration of iron

In iron deficiency anaemia, iron absorption is increased and rapid rises in haemoglobin levels are usual. The duration of therapy necessary to saturate bony iron stores may be 3 months longer than it takes to achieve normal haemoglobin levels in the non-pregnant woman. Oral therapy can be given as ferrous sulphate (200 mg three times daily) after food. For those who experience gastro-intestinal side-effects, ferrous gluconate, ferrous succinate or ferrous fumarate should be tried. Intolerance can be decreased if the dose is taken with milk or with meals. Liquid preparations are useful.

*In view of the dangers to children of iron poisoning the tablets should be dispensed in child-proof containers and mothers should be warned of these dangers.*

### Parenteral administration of iron

This may have to be considered when the patient is either unable to tolerate oral therapy, in the presence of malabsorption or when there is need for massive replacement. There is *no* evidence that it is more effective than oral iron, apart from these conditions. The two most widely used preparations are iron-dextran and iron-orbitol/citric acid complexes, both of which contain 50 mg of elemental iron/millilitre. The compound is taken up by the reticulo-endothelial system where the iron is subsequently split off for utilization. Two pitfalls to beware of are giving parenteral iron to a patient with thalassemia, in the mistaken assumption that the woman has not taken her oral iron, or to give parenteral iron to a patient who has already had adequate oral replacement. In both cases the iron-binding capacity of the plasma is likely to be near saturation and iron toxicity may occur. *Saturation or near saturation of iron-binding capacity is a contraindication to parenteral administration of iron regardless of the haemoglobin level.*

Toxic reactions may be acute or chronic. Transient reactions include headache, shivering, nausea, urticaria and fever. Arthralgia and lymphadenopathy may be prolonged. The most serious reactions are vascular collapse and anaphylaxis, which will require supportive measures including the use of adrenaline and steroids. Chronic toxicity theoretically includes the possibility of iron overload and carcinogenesis. For this reason the drugs are not recommended as a first line approach to treatment and are rarely used.

### Intramuscular technique

The dose is calculated to provide enough iron to restore the haemoglobin to normal and to provide 500 mg for storage.

$$\text{Amount required} = \frac{\text{Desired haemoglobin (13.5) - Patient's haemoglobin}}{100} \times 4000 \times 3 + 500 \text{ mg}$$

(Holly, 1958)

A less arbitrary answer is obtained if the real blood volume is substituted for the figure 4000. Blood volume may be estimated on the basis of 66 ml of blood/kg of body weight. A simpler formula which may be used to calculate the dose of iron required in milligrams is:

Amount required = 0.3 × patient's weight (in lb) × haemoglobin deficiency

A test dose of 25 mg is given on the first day. If no adverse reaction is encountered a daily dose of 250 mg is given until the total calculated dose is reached. The injections are given into the muscle in the upper outer quadrant of the buttock. Since the agent stains, it should be given by a Z technique, where the subcutaneous tissue is pulled to one side just prior to injection. Scarring of the buttocks is a common sequel to such injections.

### Intravenous technique

Circumstances in which the intravenous route seem preferable include a small muscle mass, sacral oedema or when an intramuscular injection may result in haematoma formation.

The course may be given in daily doses of 100 mg or alternatively the total dose may be given as a single infusion. However, a relatively high incidence of severe reactions has been recorded with this technique in antenatal patients (Clay *et al*, 1965) and 0.5 to 1.0 ml of 1 in 1000 adrenaline solution must be immediately available for subcutaneous injection.

## Blood transfusion

This should only play a very minor role in the treatment of iron deficiency anaemia, but may be necessary if the haemoglobin is particularly low or there is inadequate time for a response to iron therapy

(4–6 weeks required.). Transfusion should be carried out cautiously with packed cells and diuretic cover.

## Prophylaxis

Prophylaxis of iron deficiency in pregnancy is a frequent practice in many centres. A total daily intake of approximately 100 mg elemental iron during pregnancy maintains maternal iron stores and results in higher neonatal iron stores. The use of prophylactic iron does not remove the need to monitor maternal haemoglobin during pregnancy as a third of women fail to take their medication (Bonnar *et al*, 1969). In Sweden, fortification of flour with iron appears to have led to a reduction in the prevalence of iron deficiency anaemia in non-pregnant women (Hallberg *et al*, 1979) and may have similar effects in pregnant women.

# Folic acid deficiency

Surveys conducted in British industrial towns have shown that between 2 and 4 per cent of pregnancies are complicated by mega-loblastic anaemia, in the absence of folate supplements. In twin preg-nancies the figure may be as high as 25 per cent.

The clinical manifestations of folate deficiency include diarrhoea, loss of appetite and fatigue. The patient may also have glossitis. It has been suggested that there is a higher incidence of abruptio placentae, postpartum haemorrhage and premature delivery in folate deficient pregnancies (Hibbard *et al*, 1963), although this has not been confirmed (Fleming *et al*, 1975).

In spite of maternal deficiency of folic acid the infant's haemoglo-bin and folate levels remain normal. Folate replacement does not appear to benefit the healthy term infant.

## Investigation

Serum folate may be measured by a microbiological or radio-immunoassay. Microbiological assays are unreliable if the patient is on antibiotics. Serum folate measurements reflect the folate balance which falls towards the end of pregnancy and during acute blood loss. The red cell folate content reflects the folate status of individual red cells at the time of their formation. Thus measurement of the red cell or whole blood folate reflects the average folate stores over the preceding 110 days – the life span of circulating red cells. Therefore, the measurement of red cell folate is the method of choice in inves-tigations of this nature.

Diagnosis of megaloblastic anaemia traditionally requires a

marrow examination which is characterized by the presence of abnormal nucleated red cells or megaloblasts. However, this will not distinguish between $B_{12}$ and folate deficiency megaloblastic anaemia. Before commencing therapy a sample of blood must be taken for measurement of $B_{12}$ and folate levels.

## Treatment

For the treatment of established megaloblastic anaemia due to folate deficiency, large initial doses such as 15 mg a day are recommended to ensure rapid replenishment of stores. If vomiting is a feature, the initial treatment must be given intravenously. Where oral therapy is ineffective because of malabsorption, 100 micrograms of folic acid daily may be given by the intramuscular route. Folinic acid is preferable for patients on folic acid antagonists such as trimethoprim or pyrimethamine. If the haemoglobin is less than 8 g/dl or if delivery is imminent with a haemoglobin below 10 g/dl, slow transfusion with packed cells may be given following institution of folic acid replacement. Great care must be taken to prevent fluid overload and it may be necessary to use an exchange transfusion technique.

## Prophylaxis

Studies from Glasgow have shown that a daily supplement of 350 micrograms of folic acid prevents the development of anaemia (Willoughby and Jewell, 1966). Therapy is continued until 6 weeks after delivery and anaemia due to haematinic deficiency is eliminated when combined with a daily dose of 105 mg of elemental iron. The use of small quantities of folic acid in prophylaxis largely eliminates the risk of masking Addisonian pernicious anaemia.

# Combined folic acid and iron deficiency

In pregnancy there is often a combined deficiency of both iron and folic acid. Folic acid deficiency is not always associated with a megaloblastic blood film. Consequently it is important that in any anaemic state during pregnancy, when the haemoglobin concentration is less than 10.5 g/dl that serum iron, total iron-binding capacity and red cell folate and serum $B_{12}$ are measured early.

# Vitamin $B_{12}$ deficiency

A deficiency in vitamin $B_{12}$ may have several origins. (Table 11.2)
    Because Addisonian pernicious anaemia is a disorder of middle age

**Table 11.2** Causes of $B_{12}$ deficiency

| |
|---|
| Addisonian pernicious anaemia |
| Postgastrectomy |
| Associated with miscellaneous lesions of the small intestine such as Crohn's disease, blind loop syndrome and occasionally coeliac disease |
| Vegans, diet, eg such as Hindu and Sikh patients |

and usually causes infertility, it is rarely associated with pregnancy. However, occasional cases occur and this emphasizes the importance of measuring the serum vitamin $B_{12}$ level in any patient developing megaloblastic anaemia, especially if aged over 30 years.

## Investigation

A complication of interpreting vitamin $B_{12}$ levels during pregnancy is a progressive fall to values of 80–120 pg/ml, reflecting a physiological transfer from mother to fetus. However, normal values return over the first 6 weeks of the puerperium. To avoid the dangers to the fetus of radioactivity a Schilling test should be delayed until after pregnancy.

## Treatment

In any patient with a serum $B_{12}$ level less than 50 pg/ml, 1000 micrograms of vitamin $B_{12}$ should be given weekly by intramuscular injection and if after pregnancy the diagnosis of pernicious anaemia is confirmed treatment will need to be continued for life.

A maternal deficiency of $B_{12}$ results in low fetal vitamin stores and a low $B_{12}$ content in maternal milk. In breast-fed infants this may lead to a $B_{12}$ deficiency syndrome of apathy, involuntary movements, developmental regression, pigmentation and anaemia appearing between 4 and 12 months after birth. They should consequently receive vitamin $B_{12}$.

## *Hereditary red cell disorders*

During the stress of pregnancy a previously well compensated haemolytic state or thalassaemia trait may give rise to overt anaemia.

## Hereditary spherocytosis

This is an autosomal dominant condition which occurs most frequently in persons of British and North European stock. The majority of patients have symptoms of anaemia and jaundice and are diagnosed in childhood. The spleen is almost invariably enlarged. It is usually firm and non-tender. Pigment gall-stones develop in about 50 per cent of cases and cholecystitis or obstruction of the common bile duct may result.

## Investigation

The blood picture typically shows anaemia with spherocytosis, an increased erythrocyte osmotic fragility, a raised reticulocyte count and the serum bilirubin is elevated.

## Treatment

Splenectomy is practically always followed by complete and sustained clinical remission and is indicated in all patients except those who are symptom free and well compensated. It is not indicated during pregnancy, unless there is clinical deterioration of the mother. There may be some benefit from folic acid supplementation.

# Glucose-6-phosphate dehydrogenase deficiency (G-6-PD)

Infections or drugs such as primaquine may cause a haemolytic anaemia in sensitive subjects, particularly negroes and Mediterranean peoples. The haemolysis is self-limiting; older cells are destroyed while younger ones are resistant and the haemoglobin returns to normal once the older population of cells has been destroyed. The disease is important because drug therapy during pregnancy may precipitate a haemolytic anaemia. Such oxidant drugs include: sulphonamides, nitrofurantoin, salicylates, primaquine and water soluble vitamin K analogues.

## Investigation

When not exposed to the offending drugs the blood findings are normal. During haemolysis Heinz bodies and spherocytes may appear. Several screening tests are available for the diagnosis of G-6-PD deficiency. Most demonstrate the presence or absence of G-6-PD by testing the ability of the red cells to generate NADPH from NADP, a reaction which directly depends upon the availability of G-6-PD.

## Treatment

In the mother treatment is seldom necessary. However, in the neonate with G-6-PD deficiency, early severe neonatal jaundice may require exchange transfusion.

# *Haemoglobinopathies*

These disorders can be divided into two groups:

1. Structural haemoglobin variants where there is a substitution of one or more amino acids in the globin chain.
2. Thalassaemias in which globin chain synthesis is unbalanced.

# Structural haemoglobin variants

When the possession of a haemoglobin variant gives rise to a clearly defined disease the person is said to have a haemoglobinopathy. Perhaps the best known example is the sickle cell haemoglobinopathy (HbS). The sickling of red cells in the circulating blood has two major pathological effects. The distorted cells cause a marked increase in blood viscosity and block small blood vessels, impairing flow and causing ischaemia and infarction of the tissue supplied by the blocked vessels. Repeated episodes of sickling lead to red cell deformity and intravascular and extravascular haemolysis.

## Sickle cell trait

This is the carrier state of HbS and occurs in about 8 per cent of Black Americans and between 20 and 50 per cent of some African tribes. In the heterozygous state, HbS comprises less than 50 per cent of the haemoglobin in the cells which do not undergo sickling in the natural state. Sickle cell trait does not cause anaemia and is usually asymptomatic.

## Sickle cell anaemia

The diagnosis is usually made in childhood. Patients are particularly sensitive to bacterial infection with *Salmonella, Pneumococcus, Meningococcus* and *Haemophilus influenzae*. Splenomegaly is present during childhood but repeated episodes of infarction lead to atrophy. In adult life, clinical severity is highly variable, a significant number of adults are able to lead relatively normal lives, punctuated by only occasional episodes of illness. In many patients the disease is severe with frequent sickling crises. Vaso-occlusive crises give rise to sudden attacks of bone pain, usually in the limbs or abdomen. Aplastic crises occur when there is sudden cessation of marrow erythropoiesis. Haemolysis occurs and the red cell mass rapidly diminishes to life threatening levels.

Pregnancy is relatively uncommon in female patients with sickle cell anaemia and is associated with a high degree of maternal morbidity and fetal loss. Sickle cell crises and infective complications, especially urinary tract infection, are common.

## Investigation

The diagnosis is based on the demonstration of a positive sickle test or a positive haemoglobin solubility test in patients with chronic haemolytic anaemia. The screening test should be confirmed by an electrophoretic analysis.

## Treatment

There are no major antenatal problems in women with the sickle cell trait apart from an increased incidence of pyelonephritis.

*There are potential hazards due to hypoxia during general anaesthesia.*

In homozygous sickle cell disease there is a substantially higher incidence of prematurity, abortion, stillbirth, pulmonary complications and sickling crises. An inability to concentrate urine puts pregnant women with sickle cell disease at risk of dehydration. Frequent blood transfusions are necessary in the majority of such patients as pregnancy advances. Increased folate supplementation and oral bicarbonate to keep the urine alkaline are standard therapy. Overt crises are best treated by exchange transfusion (2.5 litres out; 3 litres in). An alternative policy is to give regular transfusions of 3 to 4 units at about 6 week intervals to maintain a circulating normal adult haemoglobin of 60–70 per cent throughout late pregnancy. (Huehns, 1974 and Letsky, 1976). Although prophylactic transfusion therapy reduces marrow production, folic acid supplements should still be prescribed.

During labour and delivery any stimulus to sickling such as hypoxia, acidosis, dehydration or circulatory depression must be avoided. If intravenous fluids are used, lactate should be included in the regimen; prophylactic antibiotics should also be given. *If surgery is required great care is needed to minimize sickling.*

# Thalassaemias

There are two main groups of thalassaemias, one affecting the synthesis of $\alpha$ chains and the other $\beta$ chains of the haemoglobin molecule. In $\beta$ thalassaemia, the inadequate production of $\beta$ chains leads to a reduction in the amount of normal haemoglobin in the red cell and a microcytic hypochromic anaemia. The total haemoglobin is maintained in part, by the production of $\gamma$ and $\delta$ chains and thus increased HbF or $HbA_2$ are usually found. The lack of $\beta$ chains leads to accumulation of free, uncombined $\alpha$ chains within the developing red cells and their premature destruction in the marrow.

In $\alpha$ thalassaemia the levels of HbA, HbF and $HbA_2$ are equally depressed since they all have $\alpha$ chains and there is usually a microcytic hypochromic anaemia. In the absence of sufficient $\alpha$ chains, excess $\beta$ chains or $\gamma$ chains aggregate to form Hb-H ($\beta_4$) or Hb-Bart's ($\gamma_4$).

## $\beta$ Thalassaemia minor

$\beta$ thalassaemia minor is the heterozygous state and is characterized by a moderate reduction in $\beta$ chain synthesis. The disorder is common in Mediterranean peoples, but is also found in other races. Clinically it is usually a mild disorder with little or no anaemia, no symptoms and a normal life expectancy. The spleen may be palpable. The condition is commonly not diagnosed until adolescence or adult life and may be detected first during routine haematological screening in pregnancy.

### Investigation

The main problem is in the differentiation of this condition from iron deficiency and the first suspicion may arise because of an anaemia refractory to haematinics. Haemoglobin is often normal or mildly reduced, but rarely less than 10 g/dl. The red cell count is often normal; but examination of a blood film may show anisocytosis and microcytosis. In the majority of cases there is an increase in $HbA_2$. A small increase in HbF occurs in about 50 per cent of cases.

### Treatment

The aim in pregnancy is to maintain haemoglobin at a level above which patients become symptomatic (about 8 g/dl). Five milligrams of folic acid should be given three times daily because of the increased haemopoeisis. If the haemoglobin level falls, a simple transfusion should be given to prevent intra-uterine hypoxia and cardiac failure. *Iron supplementation is contraindicated unless iron deficiency is proven.* Usually the iron stores are adequate but not utilized and excess iron could result in toxicity.

## β Thalassaemia major

This is the homozygous state. The child usually fails to thrive and is of short stature. Menarche is often delayed and secondary sex characteristics undeveloped. Pregnancy is consequently rare, but if it occurs the patient is likely to require repeated transfusions in later pregnancy.

# Thrombocytopaenia
## Idiopathic or autoimmune thrombocytopaenic purpura

This autoimmune disorder is particularly common in young women and may appear in one of two clinical forms. The first is acute and self-limiting, the other is characterized by chronic recurrent bleeding over many months or years and it is this type that usually occurs in adults. Skin is the commonest site of haemorrhage and there are often multiple petechiae or ecchymoses. Bleeding from mucous membranes may take the form of epistaxis, haematuria, melaena or vaginal bleeding. Bleeding into internal organs is uncommon, although cerebral haemorrhage may often be the cause of death. On examination, the spleen is palpable in about 10 per cent of cases; many patients have subconjunctival or retinal haemorrhages.

### Investigation

The outstanding feature is a reduction in the platelet count ranging from just below normal values to less than $10 \times 10^9$/litre. The usual associations of a thrombocytopaenia are seen with a prolonged bleeding time and a positive tourniquet test. There are few significant changes in the bone marrow.

### Treatment

Maternal complications in idiopathic thrombocytopaenic purpura are not usually severe and placental abruption and postpartum haemorrhage do not appear to be more common. However, if thrombocytopaenia is severe and associated with spontaneous bleeding, corticosteroid therapy should be tried before splenectomy. The initial dose is 1–2 mg/kg of prednisolone. It is usually followed by a prompt improvement over about 2 weeks. Treatment should be continued at the full dose for up to 3–4 weeks and then gradually reduced. Significant relapse or a failure to respond to treatment are indications for a splenectomy. This is associated with a significant maternal mortality (Hays, 1966) and surgery is best performed during the second trimester. Platelet transfusions may be required in labour or acute bleeding episodes.

The condition is frequently associated with neonatal thrombocytopaenia due to transplacental movement of the autoantibody. However, it is usually self-limiting and resolves within 1 or 2 months. It is important to be aware that it can occur in the children of women who have apparently been 'cured' by splenectomy. Because free IgG antibodies will cross the placenta the major risk to the fetus is of intracranial bleeding during delivery and consequently elective Caesarian section should be considered. In the case of a patient who has had a previous splenectomy, Caesarian section should probably be mandatory. The mother is at risk of haemorrhage from the incision and should be transfused with platelets.

Platelet counts have been done on fetal scalp samples and if the fetal platelet count is less than $5 \times 10^9$/litre prior to delivery this is a further indication for Caesarian section.

# Aplastic anaemia

Survival of both mother and fetus is rare. Usually one or other or both are lost and pregnancy should be discouraged in this condition. The disease takes two forms: one in which pregnancy supervenes in aplastic anaemia and the other where pregnancy itself causes temporary bone marrow depression.

Bleeding and infection occur in almost all pregnancies and are the leading causes of death. Patients experience symptoms common to all anaemias and include fatigue and weakness. There is a bleeding tendency due to thrombocytopaenia and neutropaenia is associated with an increased susceptibility to infection.

## Investigation

The typical blood picture is of a normocytic or slightly macrocytic normochromic anaemia with leucopaenia, thrombocytopaenia, a low reticulocyte count and an absence of immature red and white cells. The degree of anaemia will depend on the severity of the marrow depression and similarly the degree of marrow cellularity may vary from site to site. However, although a dry or bloody tap is not uncommon in most cases there will be aplastic or hyperplastic segments.

## Treatment

With the expanding blood volume of later pregnancy, repeated transfusions of packed cells will be needed. All venepunctures must be performed with careful attention to sterility because of the neutropaenia. At delivery, careful asepsis and cover with broad spectrum antibiotics are needed. Platelet transfusions should be given to cover delivery which is preferably by the vaginal route.

*Intramuscular injections and epidural anaesthetics should be avoided.*

# Disorders of coagulation

## Disseminated intravascular coagulation

Disseminated intravascular coagulation is due to the excessive production of activated factor X and thrombin in the circulation. Injury to endothelial cells is a major stimulus to the intrinsic clotting

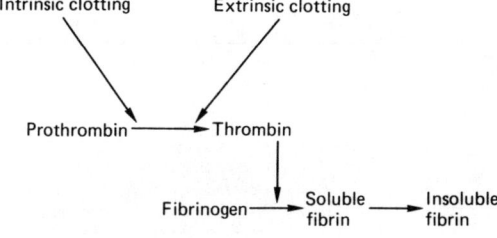

Normal clotting mechanism

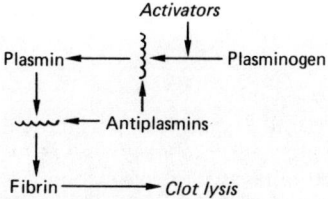

Normal fibrinolytic mechanism

**Fig. 11.1** Normal clotting and fibrinolytic mechanisms.

system and probably occurs during severe sepsis. In pregnancy-related sepsis, tissue thromboplastin may also be released. Tissue thromboplastin activates the extrinsic clotting system and is liberated by injured or necrotic tissue during abruption, retention of a dead fetus or hydatidiform mole. Disseminated intravascular coagulation from an amniotic fluid embolus is probably due to the coagulant activity of amniotic fluid itself.

Disseminated intravascular coagulation may occur in a number of obstetric complications including eclampsia, abruption, retained dead fetus, amniotic fluid embolism, saline induced abortion, sepsis, hydatidiform mole, and liver damage. Bleeding may be generalized and associated with purpura or petechiae and thrombosis or even absent.

## Investigation

The diagnosis can be made when the patient has a decreased fibrinogen level and platelet count with an increased prothrombin time, partial thromboplastin time and thrombin clotting time together with consistent clinical findings.

**Table 11.3** Tests of coagulant activity in disseminated intravascular coagulation

| | |
|---|---|
| Prothrombin time (PT) | Prolonged |
| Partial thromboplastin time (PTT) | Prolonged |
| Thrombin clotting time (TCT) | Prolonged |
| Platelet count | Decreased |
| Blood smear evaluation | Microangiopathic changes |
| Blood fibrinogen | Decreased. *The levels are usually elevated in a normal pregnancy and so a normal non-pregnant value should be questioned* |
| Fibrin-fibrinogen degradation products (FFDP) | Elevated |
| Factors V and VIII | Low |
| Antithrombin III | Low |
| Fibrinolysis | Enhanced |

## Treatment

The underlying cause should be corrected as quickly as possible and this may involve termination of the pregnancy. In many cases this is sufficient but in severe disseminated intravascular coagulation it is often necessary to replace the consumable blood clotting factors and antithrombin III and sometimes platelets. These products are best given as fresh frozen plasma or cryoprecipitate. The quantity given is empirical but should be sufficient to raise the serum level of fibrinogen to greater than 100 ng/100 ml.

Heparin is seldom used because it may cause bleeding even if the disseminated intravascular coagulation improves and in the presence of gross disruption of the vascular system as in placental abruption it may worsen the bleeding. Its anticoagulant effect is mediated by anti-thrombin III and its use should be reserved for patients with near total defibrination, but do not have gross disruption of the vascular system. Together with plasma it is administered as a constant infusion at a rate of 500 units/hour. The dose is adjusted according to the clinical and laboratory response.

In most cases disseminated intravascular coagulation reverses soon after delivery and a failure to improve suggests that the patient has sepsis, retained products of conception or underlying liver disease.

# Von Willebrand's disease

This is a dominantly inherited disorder characterized by a mild bleeding tendency, although it can be more severe and have similarities to haemophilia.

During parturition bleeding is less than might be expected as factor VIII levels increase and bleeding time becomes normal.

## Investigation

The diagnosis is difficult during pregnancy because of the increase in factor VIII, but at other times the disease is characterized by a prolonged bleeding time and a decreased factor VIII activity.

## Treatment

Factor VIII activity rises slowly until the 11th week of gestation and then remains constant until the middle of the third trimester after which it rises sharply to a peak at term. Consequently an early mis-carriage is associated with an increased risk of haemorrhage. At term, vaginal delivery is usually safe and does not require cover with factor VIII concentrate. However, if the factor VIII level is less than 30 per cent of the normal range or Caesarian section is indicated for obstetrical reasons, cryoprecipitate must be given. Levels must be maintained above 25 per cent for 2 weeks after surgery, although cryoprecipitate may only be needed for 7–8 days.

# Further reading

Talbert, L.M. and Blatt, P.M. (1979). Disseminated intravascular coagulation in obstetrics. *Clinical Obstetrics and Gynecology* **22**, 889.

Taylor, D.J. (1981). Prophylaxis and treatment of anaemia. *Clinics in Obstetrics and Gynaecology* **8**, 297.

Tuck, S.M. (1982). Sickle cell disease and pregnancy. *British Journal of Hospital Medicine* **28**, 125.

# References

Bonnar, J., Goldberg, A. and Smith, J.A. (1969). Do pregnant women take their iron? *Lancet* **1**, 457.

Buckle, A.E.R., Price, T.M.L. and Whitmore, D.N. (1969). Exchange and simple transfusion in sickle cell diseases in pregnancy. *Postgraduate Medical Journal* **45**, 722.

Clay, B., Rosenberg, B., Sampson, N. and Samuels S.I. (1965). Reactions to total dose intravenous infusion of iron dextran. *British Medical Journal* **1**, 29.

Fleming, A.F., Martin, J.D. and Stenhouse, N.S. (1975). The relationship of maternal anaemia and folate deficiency to uterine haemorrhage during pregnancy and fetal malformation. *Australia and New Zealand Journal of Obstetrics and Gynaecology* **14**, 18.

Giles, C. and Shuttleworth, E.W. (1958). Megaloblastic anaemia of pregnancy and the puerperium. *Lancet* **1**, 75.

Hallberg, L *et al.* (1979). An analysis of factors leading to a reduction in iron deficiency in Swedish women. *Bulletin of the World Health Organisation* **57**, 947.

Heys, R.F. (1966). Child bearing and idiopathic thrombocytopenic purpura. *Journal of Obstetrics and Gynaecology of the British Commonwealth.* **73**, 205.

Hibbard, B.M. and Hibbard, E.D. (1963). Aetiological factors in abruptio placentae. *British Medical Journal* **2**, 1430.

Huehns, E. (1974). The structure and function of haemoglobin: clinical disorders due to abnormal haemoglobin structure. In *The Blood and its Disorders*, p. 526, Edited by Hardistry, R.M. and Weatherall, D.J. Blackwell Scientific Publications, Oxford.

Letsky, E. (1976). Haematological disorders and pregnancy. *British Journal of Hospital Medicine* **15**, 357.

Lillie, E.W. (1962). Obstetric aspects of megaloblastic anaemias of pregnancy. *Journal of Obstetrics and Gynaecology of the British Commonwealth* **69**, 736.

Mackenzie, A. and Abbott, J. (1960). Megaloblastic erythropoiesis in pregnancy. *British Medical Journal* **2**, 1114.

Punnonen, R., Nyman, D., Gronroos, M. and Wallen, O. (1981). Von Willebrand's disease and pregnancy. *Acta Obstetricia Gynecologica Scandinavica* **60**, 507.

Scott, J.M. (1962). Anaemia in pregnancy. *Postgraduate Medical Journal* **38**, 202.

Scott, D.E. and Pritchard, J.A. (1967). Iron deficiency in healthy young college women. *Journal of the American Medical Asso-*

*ciation* **199**, 147.

Tancer, M.L. (1960). Idiopathic thrombocytopenic purpura and pregnancy: report of five new cases and review of the literature. *American Journal of Obstetrics and Gynecology* **79**, 148.

Whalley, P.J., Pritchard, J.A. and Richards, J.R. (1963). Sickle cell trait and pregnancy. *Journal of the American Medical Association* **186**, 1132.

Willoughby, M.L.N. and Jewell, F.G. (1966). Investigation of folic acid requirements in pregnancy. *British Medical Journal* **2**, 1568.

WHO Technical Report Series (1968). No. 405 Nutritional Anaemias. Report of a WHO Scientific Group.

# 12

# Autoimmune disorders

Most autoimmune disorders have a predilection for fertile women in their reproductive years and so associations with pregnancy are relatively common.

## Rheumatoid arthritis

The disease may start at any age with any permutation of joint involvement. Although the majority of patients develop the disease at the menopause or later, 2 per cent of cases have their initial attack during pregnancy and 10 per cent within 6 months of pregnancy. The disease is usually a symmetrical peripheral polyarthritis characterized by inflammation of the synovium which leads to destructive joint changes. Rheumatoid nodules are often found in the subcutaneous tissues, over pressure points and occasionally in tendons. Although arthritis is the most prominent manifestation, many other systems may be involved and the patient may develop anaemia, lymphadenopathy, splenomegaly, arteritis, pericarditis, cardiomyopathy and conduction defects, pleurisy with or without effusion, interstitial fibrosis, keratoconjunctivitis sicca, scleritis, scleromalacia perforans and amyloid.

A few patients will develop exacerbations of rheumatoid arthritis during pregnancy. However, the signs and symptoms gradually improve in the majority of pregnant patients. The improvement of the inflammatory process may be related to increased blood levels of free cortisol or to enhanced phagocytosis of immune complexes (IgG rheumatoid factors). Although joint inflammation may subside during pregnancy, the basic disease process is not permanently modified, and relapse in the first few months postpartum is common.

Specific effects of rheumatoid arthritis on the course of pregnancy are uncommon. There is no increase in the abortion or perinatal mortality rate. Involvement of the hip joints is seldom so severe as to prevent vaginal delivery. However, weakening of the transverse ligament of the atlas will present a hazard to the anaesthetist should endotracheal intubation become necessary prior to Caesarian section.

## Investigation

### Rheumatoid factor

The ability of serum to agglutinate sheep/human erythrocytes, sparingly coated with rabbit anti-erythrocyte antibody, is the basis of the Rose Waaler, sheep cell agglutination (SCAT), the human erythrocyte agglutination (HEAT) and the differential agglutination (DAT) tests. All detect rheumatoid factor of the classical IgM type. Up to 30 per cent of patients with definite rheumatoid arthritis do not have IgM rheumatoid factor but do have IgG rheumatoid factor. Four per cent of people with rheumatoid factor may have another connective tissue disorder. The main use of rheumatoid factor is in prognosis where a persistent and a highly positive titre indicate severe disease.

### Antinuclear factors (ANF)

Up to 40 per cent of patients with rheumatoid arthritis have positive ANF tests, although in low titre.

Although radiological examination can be helpful in assessing joint destruction it is not indicated during pregnancy.

## Treatment

Rheumatoid arthritis is a long and debilitating illness and the general therapeutic aim is reduction of inflammatory activity and the preservation of joint function. Psychosomatic factors are also important and may be responsible for many of the miracle cure claims including diet and copper bangles. Conventional treatment includes bed-rest during exacerbations, physiotherapy and analgesics.

### Rest and physiotherapy

Activity is important and the patient should exercise within the limits of her pain. Physiotherapy is vital and 'taking to her bed' may be disastrous for the patient, although during an acute exacerbation there is a place for resting affected joints in splints to prevent the development of contracture.

### Drug treatment

Salicylates in doses as large as 4–6 g/day are commonly prescribed but their long-term use in such doses is associated with an increased risk of antepartum and postpartum haemorrhage. Although aspirin appears free of teratogenic effects there is some controversy whether fetal death is increased by prolonged usage. During the last few weeks of pregnancy, aspirin can cause neonatal bleeding due to decreased platelet aggregation.

Indomethacin is a more potent prostaglandin inhibitor than aspirin but it may lead to early *in utero* closure of the ductus arteriosus and subsequent pulmonary hypertension and it is best avoided. Antimalarial drugs such as chloroquine are mutagenic and should not be used during pregnancy. Gold salts have been known to have therapeutic activity in rheumatoid arthritis since 1927. Side-effects include pruritus, renal damage, marrow suppression and diarrhoea but because gold salts are highly protein bound they probably do not cross the placental barrier. Experience with them in pregnancy is very limited.

Progressive disease which does not respond to treatment, vasculitis, scleritis, pericarditis, pleurisy and Felty's syndrome are all indications for systemic steroids. These lower maternal oestriol levels and this reflects suppression of the fetal adrenal gland. Acute adrenal insufficiency in the newborn is a theoretical risk of long term maternal steroid therapy but in practice this complication is very rare. An Addisonian type crisis in the mother during delivery can be prevented by appropriate steroid cover.

# Ankylosing spondylitis

Ankylosing spondylitis is an erosive inflammatory arthropathy which affects the sacro-iliac joints and the spine, resulting in ankylosis. It usually affects young men, but may also develop in women. The first symptoms are of low back pain, usually worst in the morning. The disease spreads gradually to produce an increasingly rigid spine. Ankylosis of the hip results in severe disability.

The disease may also be associated with iritis in 40 per cent of patients and occasionally cardiac conduction defects and aortic incompetence.

## Investigation

Serological tests for rheumatoid factor are invariably negative, while many patients possess the HLA antigen B27. Radiological investigation of the sacro-iliac joints and the lumbar spine should not be undertaken in the pregnant woman.

## Treatment

The whole emphasis of treatment is active mobilization as immobility leads to rapid ankylosis. Regular analgesics should be used and in pregnant women aspirin is probably the drug of choice.

# Systemic lupus erythematosus (SLE)

Systemic lupus erythematosus is a chronic multisystem inflammatory disease which can involve muscles, joints, skin, kidneys and the nervous system. It is first diagnosed during pregnancy in 10 to 30 per cent of cases.

**Table 12.1** Major clinical manifestations of systemic lupus erythematosus

| | | |
|---|---|---|
| Musculo-articular | 95 % | 1. Arthralgia with synovitis in the small joints. Aseptic necrosis of bone, especially in the hip is probably due to steroid therapy |
| | | 2. An inflammatory myositis |
| | | 3. Tendon contractures |
| Cutaneous | 81 % | 1. A butterfly rash affecting face |
| | | 2. Cutaneous vasculitis |
| | | 3. Alopecia |
| | | 4. Raynaud's phenomena |
| | | 5. Purpura |
| | | 6. Discoid lesions |
| Fever | 77 % | |
| Neuropsychiatric | 59 % | 1. Epilepsy |
| | | 2. Cranial nerve lesions |
| | | 3. Hemiplegia and paraplegia |
| | | 4. Chorea |
| | | 5. Peripheral neuropathy |
| Renal | 53 % | 1. Focal nephritis is the commonest lesion |
| | | 2. Diffuse proliferative glomerulonephritis carries the worst prognosis |
| | | 3. Membranous glomerulonephritis usually presents with nephrotic syndrome |
| Pulmonary | 48 % | 1. Most often there is pleurisy with an effusion which is an exudate (protein exceeds 30 g/litre) and in contrast to rheumatoid arthritis the sugar content is normal |
| | | 2. Recurrent atelectasis and non-bacterial pneumonias |
| | | 3. Diffuse interstitial lung disease |
| Cardiac | 38 % | 1. Pericarditis |
| | | 2. Endocarditis is a post-mortem diagnosis |
| Blood | 52 % | 1. A normochromic normocytic anaemia |
| | | 2. *Leukopaenia* |
| | | 3. Coombs' positive haemolytic anaemia |

The effect of pregnancy on the course of SLE is variable. Some surveys have shown that a proportion of patients improve while others remain unchanged during pregnancy. In addition, there have been reports of exacerbations of SLE especially in the first and third trimesters and within a few weeks of delivery. Gartenstein *et al* (1962) calculated the number of exacerbations/100 weeks at risk for non-pregnant women, those in the two halves of pregnancy and during the first 8 weeks after birth.

**Table 12.2** SLE exacerbations and pregnancy

|  | Risk of exacerbations/100 weeks |
|---|---|
| Non-pregnant | 0.91 |
| Pregnancy — first 20 weeks | 3.04 |
| Pregnancy — last 20 weeks | 1.62 |
| First 8 weeks after delivery | 6.31 |

Most maternal deaths occur in the puerperium. Maternal complications correlate closely with the presence of renal disease when there is an increased incidence of pre-eclampsia.

SLE has marked effects on the outcome of pregnancy; the spontaneous abortion rate is 20–30 per cent. The prematurity rate is reported to be 28–37 per cent and newborn children are usually small-for-dates. There is also an increased risk of fetal death late in gestation. Despite the transplacental passage of antinuclear factors, clinical involvement of newborn infants is unusual. The commonest abnormality is complete heartblock in the newborn infant and this occurs in about one third of cases. Recovery is usually spontaneous and temporary pacing is not required. Subendocardial fibroelastosis is a more rare and fatal condition.

Isolated congenital heart block in an infant indicates probable SLE in the mother and she should be investigated. It can even predate the clinical appearance of the disease in the mother.

## Investigation

### Rheumatoid factor

40 per cent of patients with SLE have a positive test for rheumatoid factor.

### False positive tests for syphylis

11 per cent of patients with SLE have a biologically false positive test for syphylis and this may be detected during the routine screening of pregnant women.

### Immunoglobulins

Polyclonal hyperglobulinaemia is present in 75 per cent of patients with SLE. IgG and IgM levels are elevated, while IgA may be lowered.

## Sedimentation rate

The erythrocyte sedimentation test (ESR) is elevated in 90 per cent of patients, but it is a poor indicator of disease activity or response to therapy.

## Antinuclear factors and Lupus erythematous (LE) cells

LE cells are found in 70–80 per cent of SLE patients, but they fail to distinguish drug and discoid LE from SLE. Antinuclear antibodies occur in 98–99 per cent of patients with SLE and are the standard screening test for the disease; although they are also seen in rheumatoid arthritis, progressive systemic sclerosis, Sjorgen's syndrome and fibrosing alveolitis amongst other conditions. A highly specific test for SLE is the presence of anti-native DNA antibodies. A rise in their titre is associated with an increase in disease activity.

LE cells have been found in the blood of infants born to women with SLE. This is probably due to the placental transfer of antinuclear antibodies and they usually disappear within 3 months.

# Treatment

SLE is characterized by exacerbations and remissions and the effect of treatment is uncertain. In most centres, patients in clinical remission with normal serum complement levels do not receive treatment. Some patients are sensitive to sunlight and will benefit from UV light barrier creams. In those who are troubled by arthritis, aspirin may be the only treatment required.

Chloroquine, an antimalarial agent, may be of use in patients where cutaneous or joint manifestations predominate and are useful in discoid LE. Although they will ameliorate the disease in 95 per cent of cases they should be avoided during pregnancy.

SLE usually responds to moderate doses of 10–30 mg of prednisolone daily. Steroids are particularly useful for acute or life-threatening episodes such as pleurisy, pericarditis and haemolytic anaemia; but afterwards the dose should rapidly be reduced to 10 mg or less daily. Treatment with steroids should be contained throughout pregnancy; this appears to reduce the incidence of antepartum and postpartum exacerbations. Steroid cover is required during labour and 100 mg hydrocortisone should be given 6 hourly.

The usefulness of immunosuppressants in SLE has yet to be established and they carry the theoretical risk of teratogenesis. During pregnancy the discontinuation of azathioprine treatment for SLE has led to exacerbation of the disease, and in those few cases of pregnant women who have received such treatment there have been no malformations of the offspring.

# Polyarteritis nodosa

Women are seldom affected by this condition which usually has an acute onset and a malignant course. Patients can present with a number of different problems including malaise, fever, arthritis, digital gangrene, tachycardia, myocardial infarction, heart failure, arrhythmias, hypertension, acute glomerulonephritis, liver failure, pulmonary infiltrates and neuropathies.

## Investigation

The basis of this disease is an arteritis which results in multiple aneurysm formation. The ESR is raised and associated with a marked neutrophilia. However, organ biopsy can be particularly useful, although the diagnosis may still be missed. Angiography can be diagnostic but is precluded in the pregnant woman.

## Treatment

Pregnancy in a woman with polyarteritis nodosa is rare and most patients have died with fulminant disease in the puerperium. Patients can develop a pre-eclamptic syndrome with subsequent death from cardiac and renal failure. Offspring do not appear to be affected by the disease.

High dose corticosteroids may be of value and if the patient survives the acute phase, she may successfully have further children.

# Progressive systemic sclerosis or scleroderma

This is a disease of unknown aetiology characterized by widespread, diffuse sclerosis affecting the skin, alimentary tract, heart and muscle. Many patients have a history of Raynaud's phenomena. The skin becomes tight and tethered around the fingers and mouth. There is often cutaneous calcification and on the face there may be telangectasia.

Oesophageal involvement results in dysphagia and reflux oesophagitis leading to stricture formation. Small bowel involvement leads to malabsorption with a 'stagnant loop' syndrome. Pulmonary manifestations include fibrosis, chest infections and pulmonary hypertension. In 50 per cent of patients, primary myocardial fibrosis results in conduction defects.

Although scleroderma affects women more commonly than men; they are usually over 40 and so association with pregnancy is unusual.

Because the disease has a natural history of exacerbations and remissions, the effects of pregnancy remain controversial but the outlook is poor if there is renal involvement. The incidence of spontaneous abortion is greatly increased and premature labour is a common complication and up to 50 per cent of fetuses and neonates may die.

## Investigation

The antinuclear factor is found to be positive in 60 per cent of scleroderma patients. However, the diagnosis is a clinical one.

## Treatment

Treatment is symptomatic and consists of analgesics for arthritis, elaborate precautions against cold exposure, skin lotions and physiotherapy. There is no place for corticosteroids.

# Further reading

Hughes, G.R.V. (1979). *Connective Tissue Diseases*. Blackwell Scientific Publications, Oxford.

Kitzmiller, J.L. (1978). Autoimmune disorders: maternal, fetal and neonatal risks. *Clinical Obstetrics and Gynecology* **21**, 385.

Pitkin, R.M. (1977). Autoimmune diseases in pregnancy. *Seminars in Perinatology* **1**, 161.

# 13

# Skin diseases

When pregnant, a woman is as susceptible to ordinary skin diseases as anyone else, but there are uncommon skin conditions which are unique to pregnancy.

**Table 13.1** Normal skin changes during pregnancy

| | | |
|---|---|---|
| *Pigmentation* | 1. | Hyperpigmentation of areolae, axillae, abdomen (linea nigra) and perineal area |
| | 2. | Chloasma which affects the face and forehead. 75 % of women developed some degree of pigmentation by the last trimester |
| *Striae gravidarum* | 1. | Thin clear cut lines of atrophy which are initially pink or violet and later become white |
| *Hair growth* | 1. | The amount of hair increases during pregnancy but is followed by excessive loss for 2–4 months — postpartum telogen effluvium |
| *Vascular changes* | 1. | *Spider naevi* 60 % of pregnant white women and 12 % of coloured women have spider naevi, which appear between the 2nd and 5th month of pregnancy. About three quarters of the lesions disappear during the puerperium |
| | 2. | *Palmar erythema* Again this is commoner in white than coloured women and usually resolves at the end of pregnancy |
| | 3. | *Granuloma gravidarum* These lesions may be sessile or pedunculated and occur in the second half of pregnancy. They disappear after pregnancy but if unsightly they may be removed with diathermy or cut off at the base |

## *Skin diseases unique to pregnancy*

## Herpes gestationis

This disease occurs in about 1 in 5000 pregnancies. It usually develops during the second trimester and tends to recur in subsequent pregnancies. Intense pruritus is followed by erythema and subcutaneous oedema. Papules, vesicles and bullae subsequently appear to involve the arms, legs and periumbilical areas. The disease may become generalized and in 20 per cent of cases the mucous membranes are involved. The lesions regress and heal to leave behind areas of pigmentation within 30 days of parturition.

A quarter of pregnancies end in spontaneous abortion or intrauterine death and in those fetuses who survive there is said to be a higher incidence of spina bifida and anencephaly.

## Investigation

Herpes gestationis is associated with an eosinophilia and an increase in urinary gonadotrophin levels. Immunofluorescent studies show IgG, $C1_q$, $C_3$ and properdin within the basement membrane zone between dermis and epidermis. Recently an IgG circulating complement binding factor (the HG factor) has been isolated.

Despite its name there is no suggestion that this condition is caused by a herpes virus infection.

## Treatment

Fluid intake and diet must be maintained and if the lesions become infected, treatment with broad spectrum antibiotics such as erythromycin will be necessary. Systemic steroids and pyridoxine may also be beneficial and in severe cases it may be necessary to terminate the pregnancy.

# Prurigo gestationis

Prurigo gestationis is said to occur in about 1 in 200 pregnancies. The onset is gradual and usually occurs after the fourth month. Small papules appear on the trunk and extensor surfaces of the limbs. The lesions are often distributed symmetrically. Itching is intense and leads to severe excoriation. The eruption clears quickly after delivery but may leave some pigmentation. The disease does not usually recur in subsequent pregnancies.

Nurse (1968) has suggested that there may be two types of this condition. In the early type the onset is between the 25th and 29th weeks of gestation and the disease has a classical distribution with very pruritic lesions. The late type occurs near to term and the papules are found along abdominal striae.

## Investigation

No diagnostic tests are available.

## Treatment

The local application of calamine lotion, oily calamine lotion or 10 per cent crotamiton lotion will provide some relief. 4 mg chlorpheniramine orally four times daily or 10 mg trimeprazine three or four times daily may also be required for symptomatic relief.

# Papular dermatitis of pregnancy

This is a very rare disease of pregnancy with a generalized distribution of intensely pruritic erythematous papules. New lesions appear throughout pregnancy, but there is rapid clearing after birth. Recurrences in future pregnancies are common. The condition is associated with a high fetal mortality and the severity of the irritation usually causes great incapacity.

## Investigation

No diagnostic tests are available.

## Treatment

Systemic steroids appear to be the only effective treatment.

# *Skin diseases frequently associated with pregnancy*

# Impetigo herpetiformis

When first described, this rare condition was thought to occur exclusively in pregnancy or the early postpartum period. It usually has an acute onset and occurs most frequently in the last trimester. Groups or rings of small painful sterile pustules appear and coalesce. They are often found in the groin and along the inner aspect of the thigh. The neck is also a common site for severe involvement; as are the mucous membranes.

There may be severe systemic complications which include high fevers, vomiting, diarrhoea, arthritis, lymphadenopathy and splenomegaly. The disease continues throughout pregnancy and although it resolves after parturition there is a maternal mortality of up to 90 per cent because of cardiac and renal failure. There is also an increase in the number of stillbirths.

## Investigation

Histological examination of the pustules will show an inflammatory infiltrate of lymphocytes, histiocytes and neutrophils around superficial dermal blood vessels.

## Treatment

The only drugs which influence the course of the disease are high dose systemic steroids and wide spectrum antibiotics such as erythromycin.

## *Common diseases of the skin and pregnancy*

## Psoriasis

Psoriasis affects 2–3 per cent of the population and may have different presentations.

1. *Guttate psoriasis.* This particularly affects young people following stress or a streptococcal sore throat. The prognosis is good and intensive therapy is not needed.
2. *Nummular psoriasis.* This is the commonest form of psoriasis with characteristically salmon pink discs and plaque lesions especially on the extensor aspects of the limbs.
3. *Flexural psoriasis.*
4. *Localized pustular psoriasis.* This affects the soles and palms and there may or may not be rashes elsewhere. Treatment needs to be aggressive.
5. *Pitting of nails and onycholysis.*

Occasionally the patient develops a generalized exfoliation involving the entire body and is at risk of hypothermia, dehydration and vitamin deficiency.

There are conflicting opinions about the effect of pregnancy on psoriasis. In most cases there is a tendency for the disease to improve, but flexural psoriasis is aggravated by friction, moisture and secondary infection as well as by the patient's increasing weight.

## Investigation

The diagnosis is a clinical one. A skin biopsy may be surprisingly non-specific in equivocal cases but can show thickening of the epidermis, an increase in mitotic basal and suprabasal cells, an absent granular layer and parakeratotic cells with nuclear remnants. Small intraepidermal accumulations of leucocytes may constitute focal micro-abscesses.

## Treatment

This should include:

1. A bath before the application of dithrolan ointment (dithranol 0.5 % with salicylic acid 0.5 % in equal parts of hard and soft paraffin). This is needed daily with very thick psoriasis and about twice weekly if the scales are thin.
2. Dithrolan should be applied accurately to the psoriasis, which thins to leave a red brown stain. The darker the stain, the greater the improvement. Scrubbing the stain off in the bath delays healing.
3. The scalp should be shampooed with 0.25 % dithranol cream daily until it is smooth and then for a further week less frequently.

This type of treatment must be continued until the skin is clear, at which stage the dithranol stain peels off to leave skin of normal colour. Dithranol should not be used in the first half of pregnancy as it is teratogenic. It should not be used within a month of topical steroids either. Steroids are clean and easy to use but they fail to clear the rash and usually are followed by a relapse.

Other treatments that are used in psoriasis include:

1. *Methotrexate.* This drug inhibits the enzyme dihydrofolate reductase which is essential for the synthesis of purines and pyrimidines and should *not* be used in pregnancy.
2. *Psoralens and ultraviolet light A (PUVA).* With the energy from ultraviolet light A the psoralen (e.g. methoxsalen) is bound by a photochemical reaction to DNA preventing its synthesis and consequent cell division. It should *not* be used in pregnancy or young people in general.
3. *Etretinate.* This is an orally administered retinoid compound related to vitamin A. It has a specific inhibitory effect on severe psoriasis and must not be given to pregnant patients and contraception must be used for a year after completion of treatment as it is teratogenic.

## Eczema

About 3 per cent of the population may be affected and characteristically they have a low itch threshold to both minor and major stimuli which results in scratching and subsequent excoriation. The skin becomes sore and may exude serous fluid, whereas in non-excoriated areas the skin is dry. During early adult life these symptoms can be precipitated by such allergens as household detergents. The disease does not appear to influence the course of pregnancy.

## Treatment

The basic principles of treatment include avoiding allergens and the use of bath oils and skin emollients to prevent dry-cracking. Topical corticosteroids are used sparingly.

## Further reading

Warin, A.P. (1981). Dermatology. *Clinics in Obstetrics and Gynaecology* **8**, 431.

# 14

# Infections during pregnancy

Antibodies developed by the mother against the majority of bacterial and viral infections are associated with IgG globulins which cross the placenta so that the child is born with passive resistance against many diseases to which the mother has been exposed. Smallpox is however a notable exception since maternal immunity offers no protection to the child. Transferred maternal immunoglobulins, in general, survive in the neonate for about 3 months, by the end of which time passive immunity will disappear.

IgM does not cross the placenta and antibodies of this class are indicative of intra-uterine infection of the infant and are important in identifying a possible viral aetiology of congenital abnormalities.

Of the more frequently encountered clinical syndromes, viral disorders of the respiratory tract appear to be of little consequence in pregnancy. Many including parainfluenza types 2 and 3 and human respiratory syncitial virus may cause mild respiratory disease in adults and are sometimes cultured from the newborn; their role in neonatal disease is difficult to define. There is no evidence that the human rhinoviruses associated with the common cold adversely affect either mother or fetus.

## *Viruses*

### Rubella

In 1941 Sir Norman Gregg noticed an association between cataracts and other ocular defects, mental retardation and microcephaly, heart disease and low birth-weight with failure to thrive in infants born to women who had rubella during the first trimester of pregnancy. The disease affects about 0.8/1000 pregnancies although the figure approaches 22/1000 during epidemics (Sever and White, 1968).

Although severe disease may occur in adults, rubella is usually a mild infection characterized by a generalized rash that may be preceded by catarrh and by enlargement of the posterior cervical lymph nodes. In up to 30 per cent of women it may be asymptomatic. The rash starts as a faint macular erythema which first involves the face and neck and later spreads to involve the trunk and limbs. The incubation period is usually 17–18 days, but extremes of 12–22 days have been recorded.

Rubella causes spontaneous abortion and stillbirth in about 10 per cent of affected pregnancies, doubling the normal rate. There is some evidence that after 8 weeks the fetus develops the capacity to limit the infection. This is consistent with the observation that if the infection is acquired during the first month of gestation, the incidence of defects may approach 50–60 per cent and such defects may be multiple. Thereafter, the incidence of malformations declines until by the 16th week it is about 5 per cent. Even if the infection is acquired after the first trimester until the 31st week, the babies may show evidence of intra-uterine infection and at 2–3 years old have grown poorly and show evidence of developmental retardation.

## Investigation

### Mother

The diagnosis of rubella in pregnancy is established by serological tests. The most useful procedure is the haemagglutination inhibition (HAI) test. No HAI antibody is detectable in women who are susceptible to rubella. It appears at the time of the rash and reaches a peak 2–3 weeks later. The antibody responsible for the complement fixation (CF) test develops more slowly and consequently sero-conversion may be detected in a mother. IgM rubella antibody appears at the time of the rash and persists for 6 weeks – thus making it possible to make a diagnosis of recent infection on a single convalescent serum sample.

### Neonate

Rubella-specific IgM can usually be detected during the first year of life and since IgM antibodies do not cross the placenta the presence of this antibody in cord blood indicates intra-uterine infection and may be used as a screening test in sickly babies or those with malformations.

## Immunization

It is essential to ensure that women are immunized before they become pregnant. All schoolgirls of 13 years of age in this country are offered vaccination and they should be actively encouraged to accept. A serological test, however, remains the only guarantee of adequate immunity, though even this may be lost in time. A history of clinical rubella is unreliable because a number of infections may produce similar rashes.

Consultations for family planning or antenatal screening provide opportunities for checking young women's immunity to rubella. It is important to realize that rubella vaccination is often unsuccessful after blood transfusion and should be delayed for 4–6 months (Watt and McGuken, 1980). It may also be less effective if anti-D prophylaxis has been given and the same advice applies.

Occasionally women who are pregnant are accidentally vaccinated against rubella but although the rubella vaccine crosses the placenta and causes intra-uterine infections no pregnancy that has gone to term has resulted in an infant with abnormalities detectable at birth (Moillin *et al*, 1976).

*Although vaccine virus appears less teratogenic than wild strains, pregnancy should be an absolute contraindication to vaccination and pregnancy should be avoided for 3 months after vaccination.*

Gammaglobulin prophylaxis appears to be of little value and does not protect susceptible women from infection. It may convert clinically visible disease into an inapparent infection and may prolong the incubation period for a few days, thus adding to the difficulties of clinical and laboratory diagnosis.

### Impact of the rubella vaccination programme

Rubella vaccine has been available in Britain for 14 years and the principal target group has been schoolgirls aged 13 years or younger. Their immunization alone has had minimal effect on the incidence of congenital rubella and any impact will be observed after the first 10 years of the programme (Smithells *et al*, 1985).

# Cytomegalovirus

About half the female population in the Western hemisphere have not been exposed to this infection by the time they reach child-bearing years and as the highest seroconversion rate occurs between the age of 15 and 35 the chances of the disease coinciding with pregnancy are high. Some 3–6 per cent of apparently healthy women excrete virus in the urine during pregnancy, although the great majority of them are asymptomatic. Most babies escape serious disease or even outward signs of infection, although infection during early pregnancy may cause abortion or congenital defects. In later pregnancy, infection can cause severe fetal disease with stillbirth. Polyhydramnios is occasionally seen. If the child is born alive it is often of low birth-weight, becomes jaundiced and has hepatosplenomegaly, thrombocytopenic purpura, choroidoretinitis and anaemia. Others will show spasticity, microcephaly and mental retardation.

## Investigation

### Mother

The complement fixation test is not a sensitive indicator of CMV infection, as there is cross reaction with other herpes virus. The indirect haemagglutination test is more reliable and there are also neutralization and fluorescent antibody tests available.

### Neonate

IgM levels greater than 180 mg/litre strongly suggest intra-uterine infection and this may be confirmed by the detection of virus-specific IgM by immunofluorescent techniques.

## Prophylaxis and treatment

Both prophylactic vaccination of the mother with an attenuated strain of the virus (Stern, 1977) and treatment of infected infants with cytosine arabinoside or adenosine arabinoside (Sever, 1978) are experimental. Although drug treatment clears virus from the neonatal urine the virus often returns when therapy is stopped. Treatment may produce marrow suppression.

# Herpes simplex

Primary genital infections with herpes simplex virus (Type II) are often painful producing ulceration and inguinal lymphadenopathy. The child can be infected during delivery. Evidence of infection occurs in the first 3 weeks of life and three forms of disease are recognized. There may be convulsions due to central nervous involvement. Vesicular lesions of the skin or throat may be found with or without conjunctivitis. In systemic disease there may be hepatitis, jaundice, hepatosplenomegaly, pulmonary disease, haemolytic anaemia, petechiae and thrombocytopaenia. The prognosis in children with localized vesicular lesions is good, although 50 per cent of them develop more extensive disseminated infection. Systemic infection is fatal in over 90 per cent of cases. Infection in early or mid pregnancy may result in a congenitally malformed infant with microcephaly. (South *et al*, 1969).

## Investigation

### Mother

Herpes simplex can be cultured within 2–4 days and wherever possible a smear for cervical cytology should be taken at the same time as the swab, since cytological changes including multinucleate cells and prominent eosinophilic intranuclear inclusions can be detected even though attempts to cultivate the virus fail.

### Neonate

In the child there will be an elevation of IgM levels to greater than 220 mg/litre during the neonatal period and specific IgG HSV antibody will be detected.

## Treatment

The only method at present available for prevention of neonatal herpes is to stop the child being exposed to the virus during delivery. When active disease is present this is usually accomplished by performing Caesarian section at 38–39 weeks. In one series, the risk of infection for the child was 54 per cent if the mother had clinically evident infection at the time of vaginal delivery. When Caesarian section was performed within 4 hours of rupture of the membranes, the risk was reduced to 7 per cent. This was increased to 94 per cent if the section was delayed beyond 4 hours (Nahmias *et al*, 1975). Caesarian section should ideally be performed before the membranes are ruptured.

Chemotherapy for congenital infection using adenine arabinoside is under investigation as are idoxuridine and acyclovir. There may be some benefit if they are started within a few days of infection but they should not be used during pregnancy.

## Varicella zoster

Varicella zoster affects 1 in 2000 pregnancies. Infection in the first 16 weeks is associated with a 5 per cent incidence of congenital abnormalities including cataracts, optic atrophy, choroidoretinitis, hypoplasia of the limbs and mental retardation (Williamson, 1975).

Varicella late in pregnancy leads to chickenpox skin lesions and severe pneumonia in the neonate. Maternal infection, 5–15 days before delivery, is associated with disease in the infant and symptoms usually develop within 4 days of birth. The infection is not usually severe because of maternal antibodies. However, if the maternal infection was only 4 days before delivery up to 30 per cent of the children develop disseminated disease which can be fatal.

## Investigation

### Mother

Maternal antibody is generally measured by immune adherence or enzyme linked immunosorbent assay (ELISA) and is present from 7 days after the onset of the rash. The antibodies detected by complement fixation do not persist as long.

### Neonate

Isolation of the virus is difficult, but may be made from vesicular fluid within 4 days of the appearance of the rash.

## Treatment

Gamma globulin given to the recently infected mother probably does not protect newborn infants. Gamma globulin should be given to newborn infants within 72 hours of birth when mothers have had varicella in the previous four days.

# Enteroviruses

## Poliovirus

Poliomyelitis continues to be a widespread, crippling disease and although now rare in developed countries with high vaccination rates, outbreaks still occur. Evidence that pregnant women are particularly susceptible has not been confirmed. Polio virus does not appear to damage the fetus, although there is a high fetal wastage during the first trimester. If contracted near term, the infection can produce disease in the newborn.

## Prophylaxis

Oral polio vaccine has been given to large numbers of pregnant women without adverse effect. Travellers, even if pregnant, outside Northern Europe, North America, Australia and New Zealand should be immunized with oral vaccine or given a booster before departure (Dick, 1978).

## Coxsackie B virus

This disease passes unnoticed in the mother but placental transmission results in myocarditis and meningitis in the infant which can often be fatal.

# Myxovirus

Mumps, measles and influenza are associated with increased fetal mortality rates, but do not seem to cause either chronic infection or congenital deformities. Abortion rates of 27 per cent have been reported in mumps (Siegel *et al*, 1966) and 33 per cent in measles (Christensen *et al*, 1953). In pandemics fetal death occurred in 40 per cent of patients with influenza and the infection may cause anencephaly (Coffey and Jessop, 1959 and 1963).

**Table 14.1** Viral vaccines contraindicated during pregnancy

| Vaccine | Possible side-effects Mother | Fetus |
|---------|------------------------------|-------|
| Measles | 1. Fever 2. Rash 3. Susceptibility to bacterial infection | Death *in utero* |
| Mumps | None | Death *in utero* |
| Rubella | 1. Lymphadenopathy 2. Rash 3. Arthralgia | Rubella-like syndrome |
| Vaccina | Encephalitis | Generalized infection |

# Bacteria

In the less privileged parts of the world infection due to *Streptococcus* continues to wreak havoc amongst mothers and infants. In a recent report on maternal deaths in England and Wales 12 per cent were due to sepsis (Tomlinson *et al*, 1979) and neonatal sepsis remains an important cause of infant mortality. Antibiotics are in common use during pregnancy and in one study 37 per cent of mothers received antibiotics at some stage (Doering and Stewart, 1978).

# Antibiotics and pregnancy

Virtually all antibiotics cross the placenta in some degree and are secreted in the breast milk. As far as is known most antibiotics are safe in pregnancy with some exceptions. (Table 14.2)

Nevertheless all antibiotics should be used only when absolutely necessary during the time of organogenesis. Having reached the fetus, the distribution of drugs is different from that in the newborn. There is shunting of blood which carries the drug away from the fetal lung. This can be of particular significance in prolonged labour when the

**Table 14.2** Antiobiotics to be avoided in pregnancy

| Antibiotic | Adverse effects |
|---|---|
| Tetracyclines | 1. Discolouration of fetal teeth<br>2. Acute fatty liver of pregnancy in the mother |
| Chloramphenicol | 1. Grey syndrome in the neonate which consists of sudden collapse at a few days old with hypothermia, flaccidity and an ashen colour<br>2. Rarely maternal marrow aplasia |
| Streptomycin | 1. VIII nerve damage in the children of mothers who received the drug during pregnancy |
| Sulphonamides | 1. Increased risk of kernicterus in the fetus |
| Co-trimoxazole | 1. Theoretical risk of teratogenicity in the first trimester<br>2. Risk of kernicterus if given in the third trimester |
| Gentamicin | 1. Ototoxic in fetus |

route of fetal infection is via liquor to the fetal lung which can allow the development of neonatal pneumonia.

## Specific bacterial infections

## Chlamydia trachomatis

During the past decade an increasing number of sexually transmitted diseases have been attributed to *Chlamydia trachomatis*, including cervicitis, salpingitis, urethral syndrome, urethritis and perinatal infection. However, in many cases there are no symptoms.

The infant born to a woman with an infected cervix has a 60–70 per cent risk of acquiring the infection during passage through the birth canal. The infant may develop conjunctivitis within 2 weeks and in up to 20 per cent of infants pneumonia may develop within 3–4 months. Transmission of *Chlamydia* does not occur *in utero*.

### Investigation

Although cytological examination of scrapings from the genital tract may demonstrate inclusions, the test is of poor sensitivity. Serology is not particularly useful as there are high background rates in any sexually active population and a raised titre may not necessarily indicate active infection. *Chlamydia* are obligate intracellular parasites and they can be cultured in susceptible tissue lines.

## Treatment

Caesarian section will prevent infection of the neonate provided that it is carried out shortly after rupture of the membranes. The mother can be treated with erythromycin. Once born by the vaginal route the neonate should receive ocular prophylaxis with erythromycin ointment.

# Gonorrhoea

Although asymptomatic gonorrhoea can often present as an acute urethritis, infection of the cervix may also occur. From the initial site of infection the organisms may spread to infect Bartholin's glands, uterus, oviducts, ovaries and peritoneum. Invasion of the blood may occasionally cause infection of the joints and tendon sheaths and rarely endocarditis.

In pregnancy, the risk of developing disseminated infections may be increased with the possibility of miscarriage, intra-uterine death and gonococcal amnionitis which can be lethal to the fetus, but this is quite rare. Gonococcal ophthalmia neonatorum is acquired during birth.

## Investigation

Although there are many diagnostic tests the best clinical test is the Gram smear, in which films of pus are examined for Gram-negative intracellular diplococci. As the infection continues the diagnosis becomes more difficult and it is essential to attempt to culture the organisms.

## Treatment

Antibiotic treatment should be with penicillin.

# Syphylis

The primary chancre appears 9–90 days after infection usually on the genitalia. It may pass unnoticed in women and the absence of symptoms does not exclude infection. The secondary stage occurs 6–12 weeks later and takes the form of rashes and erosions of the mucous membranes. For up to 2 years after infection the woman may still develop moist lesions of the mucous membranes which are infective. During this period the woman is highly infectious to her fetus. The tertiary stage is often delayed for several years and is characterized by chronic inflammatory lesions (gummata) or neurological degeneration which may take the form of tabes dorsalis or general paralysis of the insane. Infectivity to the fetus continues for some years getting progressively less with time until it ceases about 9 years after the initial infection.

It was formerly thought that *Treponema pallidum*, the causative organism of syphylis, could not cross the placenta until 20 weeks. This is now thought to be wrong and the fetus can be infected at any stage. A close temporal syphylitic infection to pregnancy increases the risk of fetal infection. If the infection is overwhelming and the fetus has time to develop the disease before delivery, late miscarriage may occur. If it is not severe enough to cause fetal death the child may be born with clinical syphylis or develop it any time from birth to early adult life.

## Investigation

Routine antenatal screening tests for syphylis should include FTA-ABS (Fluorescent treponemal antibody, absorbed) which is the most sensitive serological test for syphylis and the first to become positive in the course of infection. If the infection is at a late stage TPHA (*Treponema pallidum* haemagglutination) should be performed as well. Reagin tests which include the classical complement fixation test (Wasserman reaction) and flocculation test (Kahn reaction) are non-specific and become negative in late infection. The availability of these tests will vary from one laboratory to another.

Positive serological tests for syphylis can be due to technically false positive or biologically false positive reactions. Technical errors in labelling may be excluded by repeating the test. Biologically false positives may be due to systemic lupus erythematosus, rheumatoid arthritis, malaria or even herpes.

## Treatment

Most women with syphylis discovered in pregnancy will have clinically latent disease. Because of the pregnancy it is reasonable to omit a lumbar puncture. Accordingly these patients should be treated with a dose of penicillin adequate to cure neurological involvement if present. This consists of 600 000 units of procaine penicillin G daily for 17 days by intramuscular injection. If there is any suggestion that the patient may be unable or unwilling to follow this regime, longer acting preparations such as benzathine penicillin may be used. For patients sensitive to penicillin, erythromycin stearate for 2 to 3 weeks is the alternative and this should be given intravenously to ensure placental transfer.

The newborn child should receive 150 000 units of procaine

penicillin G daily for 10 to 15 days after birth. If there is gross disease with hepatic enlargement it is necessary to consider systemic steroids 24 hours before penicillin and continued for the first 48 hours of treatment to prevent a Herxheimer reaction consisting of fever, myalgia and tachycardia due to release of endotoxin.

The patient's husband or sexual partner must be investigated and if infected, treated.

# Typhoid fever

The onset of typhoid fever is insidious with a stepwise increase in temperature over 4 or 5 days. The pulse is relatively slow for the degree of pyrexia. Malaise, headache and aching limbs are common at this stage. At the end of the first week, a rash may appear on the abdomen and back consisting of 'rose spots' which fade on pressure. At about 7–10 days splenomegaly is present and diarrhoea appears. If the patient is not treated she will deteriorate and develop septicaemia and may perforate and die during the third week of the illness.

Early reports, prior to the advent of effective antibiotic therapy, recorded a 'relative bradycardia' in both mother and fetus. There was an increased maternal mortality with premature labour and spontaneous abortion. Even with present antibiotic therapy it is possible for the infection to spread to the fetus *in utero* or at birth. This can cause fetal liver necrosis.

## Investigation

During the first week of the infection, blood culture is especially important as the organism is absent from the faeces.

The earliest serological response is a rise in the titre of the O antibody (somatic); H antibody (flagella) develops more slowly and persists longer. During the second week the Widal agglutination reaction becomes positive, but often at low titre.

## Treatment

The antibiotic of choice is chloramphenicol, but because of fetal toxicity it should be avoided in pregnancy and ampicillin should be used in a dose of 1 g, 6 hourly for 2 weeks.

# *Protozoa*

# Malaria

Malaria is prevalent in the Tropics and to a lesser extent the sub-tropics. The growth of international travel has resulted in an increase in the number of cases imported to Western Europe and North America.

## Plasmodium vivax, ovale and malariae malaria

Less than 1 per cent of the red cells are parasitized so the pathological and clinical effects are seldom severe and death is uncommon. Fever of up to 40°C is recorded and may be intermittent in a tertian (alternate days) or quartan (every third day) manner. The typical sequence is a cold stage associated with rigors, followed by a hot stage with the fever peaking, to be followed by a sweating stage. In mild infections, the symptoms may be much less prominent, especially in indigenous peoples with a high degree of immunity.

## Plasmodium falciparum malaria

Features vary from asymptomatic light parasitaemia to a rapidly fatal infection with a high parasitaemia. Fever may be high (41°C) and is often continuous. In some patients, the temperature is normal or low. Other symptoms include headache, abdominal pain, dizziness, vomiting and diarrhoea.

On examination, orthostatic hypotension, tender enlargement of the liver, jaundice and anaemia are often found. Splenomegaly is variable in the first few days. Cerebral features include delirium, psychosis, convulsions and coma. During pregnancy, mothers living in endemic areas may experience a marked breakdown in their immunity especially during the second trimester. Haemolytic crises may occur and the pregnancy may end in abortion or prematurity and impaired fetal growth (Jelliffe, 1967).

## Investigation

The common microscopic characteristics of falciparum malaria include a high concentration of parasites, a predominance of thin-shaped trophozoites, more than one ring in some red cells and the presence of sausage-shaped gametocytes. The other malarias typically cause a low concentration of parasites. The asexual rings tend to be thicker and amoeboid forms are common.

## Treatment

No antimalarial drug is entirely safe in pregnancy. Pyrimethamine and proguanil are folate antagonists and should be avoided, if possible, during the first trimester although there is no evidence that either is teratogenic in the doses used for malaria. It is wise to give 15 mg of calcium folinate as a daily supplement (Trussel and Bexley, 1981). Chloroquine is suspected of causing neonatal deafness when used in the first trimester but the evidence for this is poor and it is safer than quinine. Dapsone and primaquine produce haemolysis in patients with glucose-6-phosphate dehydrogenase deficiency and may do so in neonates even without this deficiency.

Residents of an endemic area already taking antimalarial drugs should continue to take them during pregnancy. Residents who become pregnant but do not normally take antimalarials should be given an initial therapeutic dose to clear any pre-existing parasitaemia (eg. chloroquine 600 mg) and this should be followed by a regular prophylaxis until 6 weeks after confinement. The resulting drop in immunity is temporary and not dangerous, although reinfection may be clinically apparent (Lawson and Stewart, 1967).

**Table 14.3** Malaria prophylaxis

---

*Chloroquine sensitive areas*
1.  100–200 mg proguanil daily
2.  300 mg chloroquine daily
3.  25 mg pyrimethamine daily

*Chloroquine resistant areas*
1.  Fansidar (500 mg sulphadoxine and 25 mg pyrimethamine) once weekly
2.  Maloprim (12.5 mg pyrimethamine and 100 mg dapsone) once weekly

Prophylaxis is provided by *one* of the above drugs.

---

Visitors to an area where malaria is endemic, should take prophylactic medication throughout their stay and for 6 weeks after their return, or for the duration of the pregnancy, whichever is longer.

The acute attack is treated with an intravenous infusion of 5–10 mg/kg of chloroquine every 12–24 hours. Each dose is given as a 4 hour intravenous infusion. After three doses a further few doses should be given orally so that the total dose is 50 mg/kg. If clinical improvement does not occur in the first 5 hours quinine should be substituted for chloroquine. The usual dose of quinine is 5–10 mg/kg infused slowly over 4 hours. The interval between doses should be 12–24 hours. Usually four doses will bring the disease under control and oral therapy with a single dose of Fansidar will achieve a complete cure.

# Toxoplasmosis

This disease has a worldwide distribution, but is most frequently seen in the Tropics. In its acquired form, it is a disease of children and young adults. Many cases are not recognized clinically, but in some there is an acute onset with fever, muscular weakness and fatigue, with painless enlargement of the lymphatic glands in the cervical chain. If this occurs during pregnancy the fetus may develop congenital toxoplasmosis which affects between 1 in 4000 and 1 in 14 000 live births. The infant may be jaundiced and have hepatomegaly. Choroidoretinitis, hydrocephalus and cerebral calcification may also occur. Abortion, stillbirth or severe congenital disease can follow infection early in pregnancy. The fetus is not affected by any infection acquired prior to pregnancy as it is protected by the transplacental passage of maternal antibody. Thus women giving birth to an affected child in one pregnancy will not normally have problems in subsequent pregnancies.

## Investigation

The diagnosis depends upon serology. The dye test is used to demonstrate antibodies in rising titres. To discount the effect of passively transferred maternal antibodies, only titres of 256 or higher are significant in children suspected of having congenital disease. An infection is commonly subclinical it will only be detected if routine screening for antibodies is carried out. As the disease may only affect 1 in 5000 pregnancies the cost effectiveness of such routine screening needs to be assessed and perhaps should only be offered to high risk groups such as cat owners. Women with an initial negative antenatal test should be tested again during pregnancy and seroconverters treated.

## Treatment

1 mg/kg body weight of pyrimethamine (up to a maximum of 75mg) every 24 hours with 1 g of sulphadiazine every 6 hours should be given for 14 days. Because of the large dose of pyrimethamine required it should be avoided in the first trimester because of folate antagonism. Sulphadiazine should be avoided near term because of the risk of hyperbilirubinaemia and kernicterus in the neonate.

# Worm infestations

**Table 14.4** Worm infestations during pregnancy

| Worm | Major clinical effect | Treatment and effect on pregnancy |
|---|---|---|
| Schistosomiasis | 1. Tissue destruction may interfere with vaginal delivery<br>2. Gastro-intestinal or genitourinary disease are major clinical manifestations | Treatment should be delayed until after pregnancy as drugs are toxic |
| Hookworm | 1. Significant anaemia due to blood loss which correlates with the degree of infestation | Mild infestations should be treated with iron replacement. In heavy infestations a single dose of 5 g of Pephenium is effective in *Ankylostoma duodenale* but must be given on 3 successive mornings for *Necator americanus*. Recurrence is common in the puerperium |
| Whipworm | Chronic diarrhoea and blood loss | None until after pregnancy as mebendazole is teratogenic |
| Tapeworm | 1. Increased appetite<br>2. Dyspepsia and colic | Treatment can probably be delayed until after pregnancy. A single dose of 2 g of niclosamide is effective and safe |
| Roundworm | 1. In larval phase there may be wheezing and haemoptysis<br>2. Adult worms may obstruct hollow organs and lead to severe disease | Treatment during pregnancy should be restricted to women with a heavy infection. A single dose of 4 g piperazine at night may be used. As present there is no evidence of teratogenicity |

# Further reading

Buttigieg, G. (1985). Detection and management of syphylis in pregnancy. *British Journal of Hospital Medicine* **33**, 28.

Dick, G.W.A. (1978). *Immunisation*. Update Books, London.

Hurley, R. (1974). Viral disease in pregnancy. *British Journal of Hospital Medicine* **12**, 86.

Sever, J.L. (1978). Viral infections in pregnancy. *Clinical Obstetrics and Gynecology* **21**, 477.

Trussel, R.R. and Beeley, L. (1981). Infestations. *Clinics in Obstetrics and Gynaecology* **8**, 333.

# References

Ch'ien, L.T., Whitley, R.J., Nahmias, A.J., Lewin, E.B., Linneman, C.C., Frankel, L.D., Bellanti, J.A., Buchanan, R.A. and Alford, C.A. (1975). Antiviral chemotherapy and neonatal herpes simplex virus infection. A pilot study experience with adenine arabinoside (ARA – A). *Pediatrics* **55**, 678.

Christensen, P.E., Schmidt, H., Bang, H.O., Anderson, V., Jordal, B. and Jensen, O. (1953). Epidemic of measles in Southern Greenland. *Acta Medica Scandinavica* **144**, 430.

Coffey, V.P. and Jessop, W.J.E. (1959). Maternal influenza and congenital deformities – a prospective study. *Lancet* **2**, 935.

Coffey, V.P. and Jessop, W.J.E. (1963). Maternal influenza and congenital deformities. A follow-up study. *Lancet* **1**, 748.

Diosi, P., Babuscaeuc, L., Nevinglovschi, O. and Kun-Stoicu, G. (1967). Cytomegalovirus infection associated with pregnancy. *Lancet* **2**, 1063.

Doering, P. and Stewart, R. (1978). The extent and character of drug consumption during pregnancy. *Journal of the American Medical Association* **239**, 843.

Dudgeon, J.A. (1967). Maternal rubella and its effect on the foetus. *Archives of Diseases in Childhood* **42**, 110.

Duff, P. (1983). Typhoid fever on an obstetrics-gynecology service. *American Journal of Obstetrics and Gynecology* **145**, 113.

Gregg, N.M. (1941). Congenital cataract following German measles in mother. *Transactions of the Ophthalmological Society of Australia* **3**, 35.

Jelliffe, E.F.P. (1967). Placental malaria and foetal growth failure. In *Nutrition and Infection*. Edited by Nicol Aysen. R. Churchill, London.

Juel-Jensen, B.E. and MacCallum, F.O. (1972). *Herpes Simplex, Varicella and Zoster*. Heinemann Medical Books, London.

Lawson, J.B. and Stewart, D.B. (1967). *Obstetrics and Gynaecology in the Tropics*. Edward Arnold, London

Levine, M.M., Edsall, G. and Bruce-Chwatt, L.J. (1974). Live virus vaccines in pregnancy: risks and recommendations. *Lancet* **2**, 34.

McCracken, G.H., Shinefield, H.R., Cobb, K., Rausen, A.R., Dische, M.R. and Eichenwald, H.F. (1969). Congenital cytomegalic inclusion disease. A longitudinal study of 20 patients. *American Journal of Diseases of Children* **111**, 522.

Modlin, J.F., Herrmann, K., Branding-Bennett, A.D., Eddins, D.L. and Hayden, G.F. (1976). Risks of congenital abnormality after inadvertent rubella vaccination of pregnant women. *New England Journal of Medicine* **294**, 972.

Nahmias, A.J., Visintine, A.M., Reiner, C.B., Del Blond, I., Shore, S.H. and Starr, S.E. (1975). Herpes simplex virus infection of the fetus and newborn. In *Infection of the Fetus and Newborn*. Edited by Krugman, S. and Gershorn, A.A. Arliss, New York.

Public Health Laboratory Service (1970). Studies on the effect of immunoglobulins on rubella in pregnancy. *British Medical Journal* **2**, 497.

Riggall, F., Salkind, G. and Spellacy, W. (1974). Typhoid fever in pregnancy. *Obstetrics and Gynecology* **44**, 117.

Sever, J.L., Huebner, R.J., Castellano, G.A. and Bell, J.A. (1963). Serologic diagnosis 'en masse' with multiple antigens. *American Review of Respiratory Diseases* **88**, Supplement 342.

Sever, J.L. and White, L.R. (1968). Intrauterine viral infection. *Annual Review of Medicine* **19**, 471.

Siegel, M. and Greenberg, M. (1955). Incidence of poliomyelitis in pregnancy *New England Journal of Medicine* **253**, 841.

Smithells, R.W., Sheppard, S., Holzel, H. and Dickson, A. (1985). National Congenital Rubella Surveillance Programme, 1 July 1971–30 June 1984. *British Medical Journal* **291**, 40.

Siegel, M. and Greenberg, M. (1965). Poliomyelitis in pregnancy: effect on fetus and newborn infant. *Journal of Pediatrics* **49**, 280.

South, M.A., Tompkins, W.A.F., Morris, C.R. and Rawls, W.E. (1969). Congenital malformation of the central nervous system associated with genital type 2 herpes virus. *Journal of Pediatrics* **75**, 3.

Special Advisory Committee on Oral Polio Vaccines (1964). Oral poliomyelitis vaccines. *Journal of the American Medical Association* **190**, 49.

Stark, J. (1969). Respiratory viruses. *British Journal of Hospital Medicine* **2**, 1781.

Stern, H. (1977). Cytomegalovirus vaccine: justification and problems. In *Recent Advances in Clinical Virology*. Edited by Waterson, A.P. Churchill Livingstone, London.

Tompkinson, J., Turnbull, A., Robson, C., Cloak, E. *et al*. (1979). Report on Confidential Enquiry into Maternal Deaths in England and Wales, 1973–1975.

Watt, R.W. and McGucken, R.B. (1980). Failure of rubella immunisation after blood transfusion: birth of congenitally infected infant. *British Medical Journal* **281**, 977.

Williamson, A.P. (1975). The varicella zoster virus in the etiology of severe congenital defects. *Clinical Pediatrics* **14**, 553.

# 15

# Neurological disorders in pregnancy

Few neurological problems are unique to pregnancy; their occurrence in the pregnant woman may lead to difficulties in management and delivery and in particular, worry about the possible teratogenic effect of drugs used in their control. Some anticonvulsants increase the incidence of cardiac and neurological abnormalities in the babies of mothers with epilepsy. The disability associated with many neurological disorders may impair the ability of the mother to rear her child. In particular the stress and anxiety associated with pregnancy and child rearing may be associated with a relapse of multiple sclerosis.

## Epilepsy

The clinical syndrome of epilepsy represents the effects of recurrent bursts of abnormal electrical impulses from the brain. The site and type of discharge account for different forms of epilepsy.

### Petit mal

In this condition recurrent brief attacks of loss of awareness or vacancy occur and are associated with a characteristic electroencephalogram (EEG) pattern of three per second spike and wave discharges over both frontal lobes. The symptoms may resolve in adolescence or be accompanied by grand mal attacks.

### Grand mal

The onset of a fit is often associated with a characteristic aura which varies from patient to patient and is followed by loss of consciousness and tonic spasm of the muscles. Spasms of respiratory muscles may prevent breathing for up to a minute. Sustained tonic contraction gives way to sharp, interrupted jerks – the clonic phase – during which the patient may be incontinent or bite her tongue. Following the fit the patient is unconscious for a variable period and sleeps for several hours. The EEG is not characteristic between attacks and the diagnosis is clinical.

## Temporal lobe epilepsy

In this form of epilepsy patients experience sensory hallucinations, particularly of smell or taste and occasionally elaborate disorders of perception of time or place (déjà vu). The EEG shows a discharge of sharp waves or spikes over the temporal area.

## Status epilepticus

Epilepsy can be complicated by the development of status epilepticus which consists of repeated major fits without recovery of consciousness between the attacks. Status epilepticus may be associated with a lapse of treatment, but whatever its cause, treatment is required urgently as the condition carries a mortality of 10 per cent or more.

# The effect of pregnancy on epilepsy

The influence of pregnancy on epilepsy is variable. A review of 153 pregnancies in 59 epileptic patients showed that fit frequency increased in 45 per cent, declined in 5 per cent and remained unchanged in 50 per cent (Knight and Rhind, 1975). Fits tended to increase during the first trimester and alterations in therapy did not achieve better control. After delivery the frequency of fits returned to the previous pattern. Epileptic women with frequent fits (more than once a month) were more likely to have even more fits in pregnancy.

Epileptic attacks may occur during pregnancy despite freedom from attacks over many years. Indeed epilepsy can present for the first time in pregnancy, which may make its distinction from eclampsia, cerebral tumour or venous sinus thrombosis difficult.

Status epilepticus is unusual in pregnancy but when it occurs may be fatal. Usually status epilepticus develops after a series of increasingly serious fits which have failed to respond to anticonvulsant therapy. With respect to pregnancy, the longer the delay in beginning effective treatment, the more likely is the woman to go into premature labour.

## Treatment

The woman with epilepsy should not be discouraged from pregnancy unless she has very frequent fits which are particularly difficult to control, or her general condition would prevent her from undertaking parental responsibilities. Regular monitoring of plasma anticonvulsant levels is of value; the daily dose being increased to maintain plasma levels in the therapeutic ranges. There are two main mechanisms which affect therapeutic activity. During pregnancy, the volume of distribution of anticonvulsant drugs is increased and the serum levels may be lowered. Plasma protein binding can be reduced and this increases the proportion of active drug available. Subsequent dose adjustment in the puerperium may be necessary.

The object of treatment is complete abolition of seizures. However, some patients prefer partial control to an effective but unpleasantly heavy dosage of anticonvulsants. Once a drug has been chosen the dose should be increased until control is obtained or until there is danger of toxicity. Combinations of drugs are best avoided until absolutely necessary. In general, petit mal is probably best first treated with sodium valproate, grand mal with phenobarbitone or phenytoin and temporal lobe epilepsy with carbamazepine.

**Table 15.1** Therapeutic levels of various anticonvulsant drugs*

| Drug | Serum level pg/ml | pmol/litre |
|---|---|---|
| Phenytoin | 10–25 | 40–100 |
| Phenobarbitone | 15–40 | 65–170 |
| Primidone | 22–55 | 115–250 |
| Carbamazepine | 4–10 | 17–42 |
| Ethosuximide | 40–120 | 285–850 |
| Sodium valproate | 50–100 | 350–700 |

* The suitability of these agents in pregnancy is discussed in the text.

The incidence of malformations appears to be increased amongst the children of epileptic mothers on anticonvulsant drugs compared with untreated women with epilepsy, but is raised above normal in both groups (Annegers *et al*, 1974). Congenital heart disease and cleft lip palate are the more common abnormalities. Phenytoin and to a lesser extent phenobarbitone are implicated. The combination of both drugs is more likely to produce malformations than either drug used alone. The danger of congenital malformations due to treatment is outweighed by the possible harm to mother or child of uncontrolled fits. However, it is preferable to use an anticonvulsant with low teratogenicity in women of child bearing age.

Newborn infants of mothers receiving phenobarbitone may have coagulation defects similar to that produced by vitamin K deficiency with a decrease in factors II, VII, IX and X (Mountain *et al*, 1970 and Bleyer and Skinner, 1976). Bleeding may occur at unusual sites such as the pleural or abdominal cavities. It may be controlled by parenteral vitamin K$_1$ and it would seem prudent to extend its prophylactic use eg. by giving it to the mother for the last month of pregnancy, as haemorrhage in the neonate may occur during labour. It would also be of value to measure the prothrombin time of cord blood in children of mothers taking anticonvulsants.

Sodium valproate has been used increasingly in patients with petit mal. It has been shown to be teratogenic in rodents in doses much higher than the therapeutic range. A number of separate cases of women who have unwittingly used the drug throughout pregnancy have now been reported. Offspring may show a transient secondary hyperglycinaemia in the neonatal period which can cause a false positive finding on metabolic screening for aminoacidaemia in newborn babies. There are reports of an association between maternal exposure to valproic acid and the birth of children with spina bifida. Cases of multiple congenital abnormalities have been reported and the drug is best avoided in early pregnancy.

## Treatment of status epilepticus during pregnancy

Ten mg of intravenous diazepam followed by an infusion of 100 mg diazepam in 500 ml of N saline given over 2.5–5 hours should control fits. Short term use of doses up to 30 mg is unlikely to have deleterious effects, except, perhaps, in infants at risk. However, diazepam and its metabolites are only slowly metabolized by neonates and following its use during the last weeks of pregnancy sufficient drug may be present in the neonate to produce hypotonia and drowsiness lasting up to 2 weeks. If status epilepticus persists, chlormethiazole may be used as an intravenous infusion of a 0.8 per cent solution. The patient will respond quickly to any change in dosage.

# Migraine

A classical attack of migraine often begins with visual disturbance (teichopsia) which may be associated with hemianaesthesia and in severe attacks hemiparesis. The headache is usually one sided over the temple or eye. It increases in intensity and acquires a throbbing character. It is usually made worse by light and movement and can persist for days.

Migraine may show considerable improvement during the first trimester of pregnancy but in a few patients it gets worse. It has been suggested that failure to obtain relief from migraine during pregnancy implies a predisposition to pre-eclampsia (Rotton *et al*, 1959).

## Treatment

Most migraine headaches respond to aspirin or paracetamol but ergo-tamine which is often used as an inhaler is contraindicated in the pregnant patient because it induces the uterus to contrast. The use of clonidine in the first trimester is not recommended. Pizotifen may be used prophylactically to prevent migraine attacks and no adverse effects have been described in pregnancy. Propranol has been similarly used (for side-effects see Chapter 1).

# Occlusive cerebrovascular disease

Intracranial thrombosis during pregnancy is an unusual complication occurring about once in 5000 to 10 000 pregnancies. However, strokes are more common in pregnant women than age-matched non-pregnant controls and mortality is higher. Although strokes during pregnancy are often attributed to intracranial venous thrombosis; one survey has shown that two-thirds of non-haemorrhagic hemiplegias in pregnancy are due to major arterial occlusion (Jennett and Cross, 1967). For therapeutic reasons it is important to distinguish between arterial and venous thrombosis by computerized axial tomography (CT) scanning or even angiography.

# Intracranial arterial thrombosis

The onset is abrupt. The illness tends to occur in the second half of pregnancy with an abrupt onset of headache and a neurological deficit. Convulsions occur less frequently than with venous obstruction. A thrombosis may develop on a pre-existing atheromatous plaque or occlusion may be due to an embolus.

## Investigation

The neurological disorder and its underlying arterial pathology should be investigated with CT scanning or possibly in the future by nuclear magnetic resonance.

## Treatment

Anticoagulants are contraindicated. Convulsions should be controlled with intravenous diazepam or phenytoin. Physiotherapy is useful during recovery from the paresis.

Vaginal delivery is preferable to Caesarian section unless it is specifically contraindicated. Any form of analgesia will lower the blood pressure and this includes epidural anaesthesia. However, pre-hydration followed by epidural anaesthesia is the most effective way of dealing with this problem.

# Intracranial venous thrombosis

Thrombosis of the cerebral cortical veins or dural sinuses is an unusual complication of pregnancy or the puerperium. It may occur throughout pregnancy, but particularly in its later stages and is often associated with abortion or stillbirth.

The initial symptoms include vomiting, drowsiness, speech disturbance and headache. Focal or generalized fits occur and hemiparesis of gradual onset is common. The arm is affected more commonly than the leg. On examination, signs of meningeal irritation due to subarachnoid bleeding consequent upon cortical infarction may occur. When the superior sagittal sinus is affected papilloedema can occur. A third of patients die, survivors may have a recurrence later in the same pregnancy, in the puerperium or in subsequent pregnancies.

## Investigation

The diagnosis should be confirmed by CT scanning.

## Treatment

Anticoagulants are used but there is considerable risk of haemorrhage in the brain or from the uterus. The patient benefits from anticonvulsants and measures intended to lower the intracranial pressure such as methyl prednisolone. Unless there is a contraindication to vaginal delivery, labour can be allowed to commence spontaneously and delivery assisted with forceps. However, if the thrombosis occurs shortly before or during labour, Caesarian section may be necessary.

# Intracranial (subarachnoid) haemorrhage

Haemorrhage into the subarachnoid space from an aneurysm or angioma may occur at any time in adult life and is characterized by the sudden onset of a severe headache, associated with vomiting, fits and coma. Clinical examination may be normal, where others have photophobia, neck stiffness, bilateral extensor plantar responses and subhyaloid haemorrhages in the fundi. The absence of previous hypertension, oedema or proteinuria distinguishes the condition from eclampsia. Bleeding may occur with almost equal frequency in the first and second halves of pregnancy.

## Investigation

The diagnosis should be confirmed by lumbar puncture. A subhyaloid haemorrhage indicates a high intracranial pressure and precludes a lumbar puncture. For several days after the haemorrhage the cerebrospinal fluid is obviously blood-stained; it then becomes yellow or xanthochromic due to pigments formed from haemoglobin. In patients not in coma, CT scanning perhaps followed by four vessel angiography should be considered. If no aneurysm or angioma is found, further haemorrhage is unlikely.

## Treatment

Of all patients who reach hospital and receive no treatment, about 40 per cent die from the first or subsequent haemorrhage within 8 weeks. Subsequently the risk of haemorrhage is reduced. A patient in coma is at greatest risk of death and should only be investigated if she regains consciousness. In conscious patients because of the risk of further bleeds, urgent investigation is essential. If aneurysms are found in the carotid territory, surgery is performed. It has been suggested that hypothermia should be the method of choice as hypotensive anaesthesia is a theoretical hazard to the fetus. If no lesion is demonstrated radiologically, the patient is rested in bed for 6 weeks and if blood pressure remains high the appropriate hypotensive therapy is instituted. Tranexamic acid stabilizes haemostatic coagula and inhibits fibrinolytic activity. It is often used in the treatment of subarachnoid haemorrhage, although it is not of proven benefit. It has been used safely, though unsuccessfully in the treatment of placental abruption during pregnancy.

If a patient with an aneurysm recovers, pregnancy is allowed to proceed until labour occurs spontaneously and delivery may take place by the vaginal route with the aid of forceps in the second stage. Caesarian section is required if the haemorrhage occurs in the third trimester or during labour. However, if the bleed was from an angioma, elective Caesarian section at 38 weeks may prevent re-bleeding which is likely in normal labour.

If the patient with a subarachnoid haemorrhage deteriorates and it seems likely that she will die, preparations to deliver and save the child by Caesarian section should be made.

# Tumours

Pregnancy probably results in an increase in size of tumours and subsequently precipitates symptoms. The mechanism is probably one of tissue swelling as a result of fluid retention and many of the symptoms consequently resolve after the puerperium as the tumour shrinks.

## Investigation

Computerized axial tomography (CT) scanning has provided a major advance in the safe investigation of cerebral tumours, but is more limited in the investigation of spinal lesions.

## Treatment

There is no clear agreement on the management of benign intracranial tumours, but the development of a paraparesis due to a spinal meningioma calls for cord decompression. Although symptoms tend to resolve with tumour shrinkage between pregnancies, it may be advisable to consider surgical excision before subsequent pregnancies.

# Multiple sclerosis

As this condition predominantly affects young adults, particularly women, it is likely to occur in pregnancy. Plaques of demyelination and sclerosis may occur anywhere in the central nervous system and this produces a wide variety of clinical features. In the great majority of patients the onset takes one of the following forms: optic neuritis, weakness of the legs, sensory loss, diplopia or urinary symptoms. The disease often presents during pregnancy or the puerperium with urinary difficulties.

Optic neuritis begins with pain in one eye, particularly on movement, associated with progressive blurring of vision. Visual impairment ranges from difficulties in colour perception to complete blindness, but a central scotoma is probably the most characteristic lesion. The pain resolves over a week or so and is followed by a return of vision. In time, temporal pallor of the disc occurs. Weakness of one or both legs may develop rapidly and is of an upper motor neurone type with increased tendon reflexes and extensor plantar responses. Sensory symptoms usually consist of numbness ascending from the feet to the waist over a few days with subsequent recovery within a few weeks.

Deterioration of multiple sclerosis occurs in pregnancy, but the risk is small and relapses appear to be related to the 3 months following delivery rather than the pregnancy itself. It seems possible that fatigue plays a role and the mother should be advised to take as much rest as possible in the puerperium. However, if the mother is already seriously affected at the time of pregnancy, she may be so disabled within a year of giving birth that she will be unable to rear the child successfully herself.

## Investigation

Although the clinical presentation and course of the disease often leads to the diagnosis the cerebrospinal fluid is abnormal in at least 90 per cent of patients with an oligoclonal globulin pattern. This finding is not specific, but in the appropriate context it is obviously useful.

Electrophysiological methods depend on averaging electrical responses evoked within the central nervous system by various sensory stimuli. The most frequently employed visual stimulus is an alternating chequerboard pattern. A normal response is a prominent positive wave with a latency of around 100 ms from the stimulus. Although other conditions may cause delay or distortion, the technique is of particular value in multiple sclerosis as the results may be grossly abnormal in the presence of apparently normal sight. Auditory and sensory evoked potentials may be used in a similar way.

## Treatment

There is no known curative treatment for the disease. For an acute severe relapse, 40 units of ACTH twice a day, followed by a small dose for a further 1 or 2 weeks may speed remission, but has no influence on long term prognosis.

The diagnosis should not be made after only one attack because of the possibility of error. The development of symptoms and signs pointing to multiple lesions in the central nervous system confirms the diagnosis, at which stage further pregnancy should be avoided unless disability is minor. It is unlikely that the condition is directly inherited and so the mother can be reassured about her child.

# Benign intracranial hypertension

The symptoms usually begin during the first trimester. They are suggestive of raised intracranial pressure and include headache, nausea, vomiting, listlessness, dizziness and tinnitus. There may be visual blurring and scotomata and papilloedema. Signs or symptoms of a focal lesion make the diagnosis unlikely.

## Investigation

Lumbar puncture reveals a pressure greater than 25 cm of CSF. The CAT scan shows small, apparently compressed ventricles without distortion.

## Treatment

In this disorder coning does not occur on lumbar puncture and repeated puncture, lowering the pressure to normal on each occasion has been used successfully in treatment. Diuretics and steroids have also been used to aid lowering of CSF pressure. Where vision is threatened, urgent unilateral or bilateral subtemporal decompression is necessary or even a lumbar peritoneal shunt may be inserted. In most cases in pregnancy adequate relief can be achieved by use of diuretics.

# Neuropathies or peripheral nerve lesions

Any form of polyneuropathy may occur in pregnancy and compression neuropathies appear to be particularly common due to obstetric trauma, excessive weight gain or fluid retention.

**Table 15.2**  Types of neuropathy seen in pregnancy

| | |
|---|---|
| *Mononeuropathy* | *Cranial nerves* |
| *Facial nerve* | 1.  The risk of Bell's Palsy developing in pregnancy in three times greater than at other times |
| | 2.  The disease occurs particularly in the third trimester |
| | 3.  Prednisolone is of no proven value |
| | *Upper extremities* |
| *Brachial plexus* | 1.  The increased weight of breast and abdomen causes sagging of the shoulders and traps the brachial plexus between the clavicle and first rib |
| | 2.  There is often a family predisposition |
| | 3.  Treatment includes physical support and instruction in correct posture |
| *Ulnar nerve* | 1.  An isolated compression neuropathy in pregnancy is rare |
| | 2.  Full recovery usually occurs after pregnancy |
| *Median nerve* | 1.  Classically there is tingling in the medial three or four digits |
| | 2.  The tingling is usually nocturnal and painful and arises during the last trimester |
| | 3.  Symptoms are seldom severe enough to warrant immediate surgery and they usually improve during the puerperium |
| | 4.  Splints which dorsiflex the hand at night may be of value, as is local injection of hydrocortisone (25 mg) into the carpal tunnel |
| | 5.  Operative decompression may be undertaken under a ring block |

**Table 15.2** Types of neuropathy seen in pregnancy

*Lower extremities*
*Lateral cutaneous nerve of high (Meralgia paraesthetical)*

|  |  |
|--|--|
| | 1. The weight of a pregnancy and the subsequent tension on the connective tissue of the abdominal wall may lead to compression of the nerve |
| | 2. Numbness of the anterolateral aspect of the thigh occurs |
| | 3. Reassurance is appropriate as recovery in the postpartum period is common and operative decompression is disappointing |
| *Obturator nerve* | 1. Weakness of adduction may follow damage to the nerve due to pressure from the fetal head during delivery |
| | 2. Physiotherapy is the most appropriate treatment |
| *Femoral nerve* | 1. Psoas muscle haemorrhage or trauma associated with vaginal delivery may lead to weakness in extension of the knee or flexion of the hip |
| | 2. The knee jerk will be absent |
| | 3. Treatment is by physiotherapy |
| *Peroneal nerve* | 1. This may be injured if stirrups are used during delivery |
| | 2. Clinically the patient develops foot drop |
| | 3. During recovery the patient may need to wear a short leg brace |

*Polyneuropathy*
Details of neuropathies that are important in pregnancy are included in this table

| | |
|--|--|
| *Thiamine deficiency* | 1. Also known as beri beri, this disease may occur in developing countries. It is also associated with hyperemesis gravidarum |
| | 2. Paraesthesiae develop in the legs together with muscle tenderness and subsequently weakness. Untreated the patient may develop cardiac dilatation or Wernicke's encephalopathy and Korsakow's psychosis |
| | 3. Replacement therapy should be initially with 50 mg of thiamine intravenously three times a day |

*Acute postinfective polyneuropathy: (Guillain Barré syndrome)*

| | |
|--|--|
| | 1. The disease occurs no more often than by chance in pregnancy |
| | 2. The onset is frequently with mild tingling of the extremities, followed by advancing weakness of the legs. The paralysis reaches its height at 10 days which may be associated with respiratory and bulbar paralysis |
| | 3. The CSF protein is raised to 1g/litre. There is no increase in cells |
| | 4. Sudo and Weingold (1975) reviewed the management of pregnant patients with Guillain-Barré syndrome and felt that termination was unnecessary. The fetus is unaffected in mild cases. However, if respiratory paralysis developed the prognosis became grave, despite tracheostomy and intermittent positive pressure ventilation. In this situation, Caesarian section may have lowered maternal mortality |

# Myasthenia gravis

The cardinal symptom is abnormal muscular fatigue. The onset tends to be gradual and the disease shows fluctuations throughout its course. Ptosis and associated diplopia appear towards the end of the day and disappear after a night's rest. Swallowing may be difficult and speech indistinct.

The disease particularly affects young women and therefore occurs in pregnancy. The effect of pregnancy on myasthenia gravis is very variable; some are unaffected while others deteriorate. In those who deteriorate termination does not improve the mother's condition. However, there appears to be a distinctly increased risk of relapse after delivery and a puerperal mortality of 2.4 per cent has been reported (Plauce, 1964). Labour itself usually progresses normally and vaginal delivery is the rule. It is important to remember that the newborn child may transiently suffer from neonatal myasthenia and if the mother has been taking anticholinergic drugs the child will have thick tenacious secretions.

## Investigation

The diagnosis may be confirmed by the intravenous injection of a rapidly acting anticholinesterase edrophonium chloride. Initially 1 mg is given; followed by a further 9 mg if there is no adverse reaction. In myasthenia weakness will be diminished for a few minutes.

## Treatment

Several agents are available for the treatment of myasthenia of which neostigmine and pyridostigmine are the most commonly used. The treatment should be continued throughout pregnancy and the patient should be advised to take adequate rest as symptoms worsen with fatigue. Infections require prompt treatment as they predispose to relapses.

If labour is prolonged, the patient becomes exhausted and a myasthenic crisis may occur. Anticholinergic drugs should be given parenterally and the dose adjusted according to the patient's needs. The ratio of oral to parenteral dosage is 30:1. The best dose is the smallest that produces optimum strength. Failure of the patient to become stronger or an increased weakness after a dose indicates that the optimal dose has been exceeded. The term 'cholinergic' crisis is a misnomer for intoxication by anticholinesterase drugs, which cause paralysis of the respiratory and bulbar muscles. Tracheostomy and assisted respiration may be needed. Myasthenic patients often exhibit sensitivity to sedatives, narcotics and tranquillisers, and if these agents are used the dose must be reduced. Muscle drugs must be avoided if Caesarian section is contemplated.

Experience with malignant thymoma in pregnancy is limited but pregnancy possibly precipitates the extrathoracic spread of the tumour and termination is advisable.

# Restless legs or ekbom's syndrome

Some pregnant women develop deep pain in the legs, with sparing of the feet. The essential symptom is of a distressing creeping sensation in the legs which occurs at rest and is relieved by exercise. In some patients there may also be involuntary jerking of the legs. These symptoms usually appear about 20 weeks after conception and disappear soon after delivery.

### Investigation

A full blood count and serum iron measurement are important as the condition is frequently associated with iron deficiency anaemia.

### Treatment

The symptoms are usually cured by oral iron therapy; where they are not, diazepam may be of help.

# Pregnancy and labour in paraplegia

Paraplegic and quadriplegic women can successfully accept the challenge of motherhood, but pregnancy and subsequent labour do have additional complications. These include:

1. *Pressure sores*. These can be one of the main sources of septicaemia during pregnancy. The best method of prevention is the
   education of the patient and her family in not allowing prolonged pressure to produce ischaemic changes.
2. *Anaemia*. This appears to lower tissue resistance to pressure and
   reduces resistance to infections, especially of the urinary tract. If
   the haemoglobin falls below 11 g/litre, a blood transfusion is
   the quickest and safest method of restoring a normal blood
   count.
3. *Urological problems*. Renal tract infection is the principal complication of pregnancy in the paraplegic and if renal function is
   already impaired it may be wise to avoid pregnancy. Most
   patients are able to continue voiding urine until the latest stage
   when catheterization may become necessary.

If the cord is completely divided above the tenth thoracic segment, labour is painless and its onset may be difficult to diagnose and premature labour may start unnoticed. Although the first stage of labour is normal, the second stage of delivery often requires aid with forceps, due to paralysis of the muscle responsible for expulsive efforts. With lesions above T4 or T5 the symptoms of autonomic hyper-reflexia may occur during labour and should not be confused with pre-eclampsia. These symptoms include severe paroxysmal hypertension, marked diaphoresis, headaches, pilo-erection, brady-cardia and the blockage of nasal air passages. The hypertension may be associated with a marked bradycardia. (Rossier *et al*, 1964).

## Further reading

Aminoff, M.J. (1978). Neurological disorders and pregnancy. *American Journal of Obstetrics and Gynecology* **132**, 325.

Bannister, R. (1973). *Brain's Clinical Neurology*. Oxford University Press, London.

Matthews, W.B., Miller, H. (1979). *Diseases of the Nervous System*. Blackwell Scientific Publications, Oxford.

## References

Amias, A.G. (1970). Cerebrovascular disease in pregnancy 1. Hae-morrhage. *British Journal of Obstetrics and Gynaecology*. **77**, 100.

Annegers, J.F., Elveback, L.R. and Hauser, W.A. (1974). Do anticonvulsants have a teratogenic effect? *Archives of Neurology* **31**, 364.

Bleyer, W.A. and Skinner, A.L. (1976). Fatal neonatal haemorrhage after maternal anticonvulsant therapy. *Journal of the American Medical Association* **235**, 626.

Jennett, W.B. and Cross, J.N. (1967). Influence of pregnancy and oral contraception on the incidence of strokes in women of child bearing age. *Lancet* **1**, 1019.

Knight, A.H. and Rhind, E.G. (1975). Epilepsy and pregnancy: A study of 153 pregnancies in 59 patients. *Epilepsia* **16**, 99.

Mountain, K.R., Hirsch, K. and Gallus, A.S. (1970). Neonatal coa-gulation defect due to anticonvulsant drug treatment in pregnancy. *Lancet* **1**, 265.

Pedowitz, P. and Perell, A. (1957). Aneurysms complicated by preg-nancy II Aneurysms of the cerebral vessels. *American Journal of Obstetrics and Gynecology* **13**, 736.

Plauce, W.C. (1964). Myasthenia gravis in pregnancy. *American Journal of Obstetrics and Gynecology* **88**, 404.

Rossier, A.B., Ruffieux, M. and Ziegler, W.H. (1969). Pregnancy and Labour in High Traumatic spinal cord Lesions. *Paraplegia* 7, 210.

Rotton, W.N., Sachtleben, M.R. and Friedman, E.A. (1959). Migraine and Eclampsia. *Obstetrics and Gynecology* 14, 322.

Sudo, N. and Weingold, A.B., (1975). Obstetric aspects of the Guillain-Barré Syndrome. *Obstetrics and Gynecology* 45, 39.

# 16

# Psychiatric and related disorders

Anxiety in the first trimester is common. Many women are aware of the constant threat of miscarriage and those who work experience reduced standards as a result of lowered family income. Unmarried women face particularly severe social changes and stress. Unwanted pregnancy may lead to depression and attempted suicide (Hordern, 1972). The middle months are normally peaceful, although older women tire easily from the fifth month onwards so that latent depression may present. The last 3 months of pregnancy are often again, a period of anxiety and depression (Jarrahi-Zadeh *et al*, 1969). The woman may feel large and clumsy and her sleep pattern is often disturbed by physical changes. After childbirth some independence is lost leading to further emotional stress.

## Pre-existing psychiatric illness

The problems of pregnancy in patients with psychiatric illness include a consideration of the effects of psychotropic drugs and the developing fetus. These are summarized in Table 16.1. The management of pregnancy in patients who are mentally ill necessitates close cooperation between psychiatrist, obstetrician and physician.

**Table 16.1** Prescribed drugs and their effects in pregnancy*

| Drug | Use | Side-effects |
|------|-----|-------------|
| *Minor tranquillisers* e.g. diazepam | Non-psychotic depression | 1. Shortly before delivery may depress fetal and neonatal respiration<br>2. In high dose during labour may produce neonatal hypotonia and hypothermia and reluctance to feed<br>3. Metabolites probably accumulate over last few weeks of pregnancy to produce these effects even with small doses |
| *Monoamine oxidase inhibitors* | Depression | 1. Pregnancy is uncommon in patients on these agents (Tylden, 1977) |

**Table 16.1** Prescribed drugs and their effects in pregnancy*

| Drug | Use | Side-effects |
|------|-----|--------------|
| | | 2. Fatal interactions may occur with pethidine and sympathomimetic drugs (Mindham, 1975) |
| | | 3. *Withdrawal should be made gradually and 25 mg promethazine hydrochloride qds or 25 mg chlorpromazine qds given for symptomatic relief* |
| *Tricyclic antidepressants* | Depression | 1. Teratogenicity uncertain (McBride, 1972, Idanpaan-Heikkila and Saxon, 1973) |
| | | 2. Slowly metabolized by the neonate and cause tachycardia, irritability, tremor and muscle spasms (Webster, 1973) and urinary retention (Shearer *et al*, 1972) |
| | | 3. They should be withdrawn gradually and patients will require considerable emotional support (Tylden, 1977) |
| *Lithium* | Bipolar depression | 1. Teratogenic in the first trimester causing cardiovascular abnormalities (Weinstein, 1976) |
| | | 2. Produces neonatal hypotonia and cyanosis and rarely fetal goitre and nephrogenic diabetes insipidus (Beeley, 1981) |
| *Phenothiazines* | Schizophrenia | 1. Risk of teratogenicity unresolved (Rumeau-Rouquette *et al*, 1977 and Slone *et al*, 1977) |
| | | 2. Extrapyramidal symptoms in the neonate |

* ECT can be safely performed during pregnancy, although there may be an increased risk of pulmonary embolism. However, the value of ECT in the treatment of depression remains controversial.

# Psychiatric problems related to pregnancy

## Acute psychosis of pregnancy

During the last trimester some pregnant women become acutely disturbed and confused. They are withdrawn, rambling and sometimes deluded and hallucinated. The condition usually resolves with delivery of the child and appears to be a toxic, confusional state of pregnancy. Patients are often socially deprived and the condition may be a recurrence of a pre-existing mental illness or personality disorder when the prognosis is particularly bad.

## Puerperal psychiatric states

About 4 in 1000 deliveries are associated with puerperal psychosis necessitating admission to a psychiatric unit and many more women have symptoms of insomnia, anxiety and depression during the last trimester.

## Puerperal psychosis

Many women who develop puerperal psychosis have a past history of psychiatric illness and have experienced symptoms during the first or last trimester. Pregnancy and labour has often been difficult and family or marital friction is commonly seen. Surprisingly, puerperal psychosis is rare in the unmarried.

Delusions related to pregnancy, marriage and the next baby are common and strong ideas of reference, with the belief that her baby is controlled by an external influence occur. The victim may believe she has an unique understanding of the universe and life and even write this down, although the account is often confused and illegible.

## Postpartum depression

Somnolence, uncharacteristic misery, self recriminations or fears about the baby develop. Nightly chlorpromazine is of help and early discharge to caring relatives is advisable. When symptoms are severe, response to these measures is poor; the depression worsens and in-patient treatment in a psychiatric ward with mother-and-baby facilities is essential. There is a considerable risk of suicide and harm to the baby.

## Puerperal mania

In this condition women appear abnormally well and excited after delivery. They have logorrhoea, their views are complicated and interesting and their bizarre nature only becomes gradually apparent. The response to phenothiazines is poor but lithium carbonate is extremely useful. Lithium should be monitored regularly for the month of treatment needed.

## Puerperal schizophrenia

Schizophrenia presents in a spectacular way when a postpartum patient retreats from reality into her fantasy world of visions and voices. The condition may respond to chlorpromazine or a long acting phenothiazine such as fluphenazine.

## Drug addiction in pregnancy and the puerperium

With the widespread indiscriminate use of stimulant, sedative and hallucinogenic drugs the number of women of child bearing age who are physically or psychologically dependent upon such drugs is increasing. Their attendance at antenatal clinic is unreliable (Neuberg, 1970) and they often do not present until labour is established and, perhaps, compromised. The diagnosis of drug dependence is vital as an injection of pethidine or methadone may save the baby's life in an opiate dependent mother. *Morphine antagonists must not be given as they can precipitate a fatal withdrawal syndrome.*

### Heroin

Four months of regular heroin use leads to amenorrhoea; pregnancy usually occurs during a relatively drug free period. Studies of pregnant narcotic addicts have shown a relatively high rate of obstetric complications. (Stern, 1966, Claman and Strang, 1962 and Sussman, 1963). Pre-eclampsia, prematurity, placental abruption and postpartum haemorrhage are particular problems that are seen. The relative contributions of general physical deterioration, malnutrition and ill health of heroin addicts are difficult to assess.

### Treatment

Sudden withdrawal is best avoided for fear of precipitating intra-uterine death (Bewley, 1975). Abrupt cessation of addictive drugs is best attempted in early pregnancy and the mother should have her heroin intake gradually reduced and methadone substituted. Chlorpromazine and other tranquillisers may be necessary during the withdrawal.

If the patient presents for the first time in labour, pethidine or methadone are necessary to prevent distress and provide sufficient time for the infant to recover from delivery before the onset of withdrawal symptoms. The earliest signs in the mother of withdrawal include a craving for the drug, anxiety, restlessness, running of the nose, lacrimation, goose-flesh, tremors and hot and cold flushes. Later signs include aching of muscles and bone, vomiting, diarrhoea, hypertension and tachycardia. In the infant signs of withdrawal may be delayed for several weeks (Glass, 1974) but usually appear within a few hours of birth and consist of rapid respirations, intermittent cyanosis, periods of apnoea, hyperactivity and trembling, twitching or convulsions, vomiting, diarrhoea, hyperpyrexia, excessive weight loss, sneezing, perspiration and an incomplete Moro reflex. These can usually be controlled with 2 mg/kg chlorpromazine as often as is required.

## Cannabis (Marijuana)

Although cannabis has been shown to be teratogenic in animals (Epstein, 1971) its significance in human pregnancy is uncertain. A number of women who have taken Lysergic acid diethylamide (LSD) as well during their pregnancy have had babies with gross congenital abnormalities, but it is unclear whether cannabis was responsible (Tylden, 1973). Cannabis is likely to cause hypertension at the time of labour but it does not appear to affect the neonate.

## Lysergic acid diethylamide (LSD)

The evidence implicating LSD as a teratogen is conflicting. However, spontaneous abortion occurs more frequently and there is a high incidence of abnormalities in the aborted fetus. This may reflect chromosomal defects that have been induced in the parents (Neuberg, 1970).

## Amphetamines

Abuse of amphetamines is often impossible to detect but is associated with psychiatric complications ranging from severe personality changes to chronic psychoses (Lemere, 1966). There appears to be no danger in withdrawing amphetamines abruptly during pregnancy although the mothers may require considerable psychiatric support. Amphetamines are teratogenic (Nelson and Forfar, 1973) and children born to amphetamine dependent mothers may be small-for-dates (Tylden, 1977).

## Barbiturates

Barbiturate addiction has become less common in the United Kingdom. Physical dependence leads to incoherence, emotional lability and apparent psychosis. Birth leads to sudden barbiturate withdrawal for the baby and status epilepticus may ensue and even the babies of mothers weaned with small doses may be irritable, have convulsions and fail to thrive. It is extremely difficult to wean patients from barbiturates and women on large doses make poor mothers (Tylden, 1977).

## Glue sniffing

Pregnant women working in an atmosphere contaminated by volatile solvents have babies with a greater than expected incidence of congenital abnormalities, particularly anencephaly. Glue sniffers, who are addicted to similar solvents are at risk.

## Alcohol

The idea of alcohol as a teratogen is not new. In early Carthage, bridal couples were prohibited from imbibing alcohol on their wedding night in case they produced an abnormal child (Wilson, 1981). In 1900, a survey of alcoholic women in a Liverpool prison showed that children born to these mothers had an increased frequency of early fetal and infant deaths (Sullivan, 1900). In 1973 the pattern of fetal alcohol syndrome was described by Jones and Smith in Seattle. The so-called fetal alcohol syndrome occurs in the children of mothers who are moderate drinkers as well as those whose alcohol consumption is large.

**Table 16.2** Fetal alcohol syndrome (Modified from Jones and Smith, 1973)

| Clinical abnormality | Per cent affected |
|---|---|
| *Growth and performance* | |
| Prenatal growth deficiency | 97 % |
| Postnatal growth deficiency | 97 % |
| Microcephaly | 93 % |
| Mental deficiency | 89 % |
| Fine motor dysfunction | 80 % |
| *Head and face* | |
| Short palpebral fissures | 92 % |
| Defective development of midfacial tissues | 65 % |
| Minor outer ear abnormalities | 27 % |
| *Limbs* | |
| Abnomal palmar creases | 49 % |
| Minor joint abnormalities | 41 % |
| *Heart* | |
| Septal defects | 49 % |
| *Others* | |
| Slight genital defects | 32 % |
| Benign tumours of blood vessels in infancy | 29 % |

There is an increased risk of second trimester spontaneous abortion in drinkers (Harlap and Shiono, 1980). A moderate dose of alcohol in late pregnancy depresses fetal respiratory movements and drinking as little as one ounce of absolute alcohol or its equivalent twice a week may endanger the fetus (Kline *et al*, 1980). The use of alcohol to postpone premature labour is associated with fetal metabolic acidosis, prolongation of the second stage and a tendency to muscular hypotonia. Its use in this respect has waned and it has been superceded by agents such as ritodrine, which is a $\beta_2$ stimulant.

The mean birth-weight of infants born to alcoholic mothers is significantly less than that of non-drinking women. It is of note that the weight of children born to women who stopped drinking alcohol prior to their pregnancy is also lower (Little *et al*, 1980). Neonates often experience acute alcohol withdrawal with tremors, irritability and seizures. Treatment may require alcohol for the first few days of life.

## Further reading

Beeley, L. (1981). Adverse effects of drugs in the first trimester of pregnancy. *Clinics in Obstetrics and Gynaecology* **8**, 261.

Beeley, L. (1981). Adverse effects of drugs in later pregnancy. *Clinics in Obstetrics and Gynaecology* **8**, 275.

Neuberg, R. (1970). Drug dependence in pregnancy – a review of problems and their management. *Journal of Obstetrics and Gynaecology* **77**, 117.

Tylden, E. (1977). Psychiatric disorders including drug therapy and addiction. *Clinics in Obstetrics and Gynaecology* **4**, 435.

## References

Bewley, T.H. (1975). Opioid analgesics and narcotic antagonists. In *Meyler's Side Effects of Drugs* **8**, 114. Edited by Dukes, M.N.G. Excerpta Medica, Amsterdam.

Epstein, S.S. (1971). *Drugs of Abuse*. Massachusetts Institute of Technology Press, Cambridge.

Glass, L., Rodgenhowde, B.R. and Evans, H.E. (1971). Absence of respiratory distress syndrome in premature babies of heroin addicted mothers. *Lancet* **2**, 685.

Hordern, A. (1972). Psychiatric aftermaths of the 1967 Abortion Act. *Proceedings of the Royal Society of Medicine* **65**, 158.

Idanpaan-Heikkila, J. and Saxen, I. (1972). Possible teratogenicity of imipramine and chlorpromazine. Acta Paediatrica Belgica **26**, 197.

Jarrahi-Zadeh, A., Kane, F., van de Castle, R.L., Lachenbruch, P.A. and Ewing, J.A. (1969). Emotional and cognitive changes in pregnancy and early puerperium. *British Journal of Psychiatry* **115**, 524 and 797.

Jones, K.L. and Smith, D.W. (1973). Patterns of malformation in offspring of chronic alcoholic mothers. *Lancet* **1**, 1267.

Jones, K.L. and Smith, D.W. (1973). Recognition of the fetal alcohol syndrome in early infancy. *Lancet* **2**, 999.

Kline, J., Stein, Z. *et al*, (1980). Drinking during pregnancy and spontaneous abortion. *Lancet* **2**, 176.

Little, R. and Streissguth, A. (1980). Prevention of fetal alcohol syndrome: a model programme. *Alcoholism: Clinical and Experimental Research* **4**, 2.

McBride, N.G. (1972). Limb deformities associated with iminodibenzyl hydrochloride. *Medical Journal of Australia* **1**, 492.

Mindham, R.H.S. (1975). Major tranquillisers. In *Meyler's Side*

*Effects of Drugs* Vol. 8, p. 84. Edited by M.N.G. Dukes, Excerpta Medica, Amsterdam.

Nelson, M. and Forfar, J.O. (1973). Association between drugs administered in pregnancy and congenital abnormalities in the fetus. *British Medical Journal* **1**, 523.

Rumeau-Rouquette, C., Goujard, J. and Huel, G. (1977). Possible teratogenic effect of phenothiazines in human beings. *Teratology* **15**, 57.

Shearer, W.T., Scheiner, R.I. and Marshall, R.E. (1972). Urinary retention in a neonate following maternal ingestion of nortryptyline. *Journal of Pediatrics* **81**, 570.

Slone, D., Siskind, V., Heinonen, O.P., Monson, R.R., Kaufman, D.W. and Shapiro, S. (1977). Antenatal exposure to the phenothiazines in relation to congenital malformations, perinatal mortality rate, birth weight and intelligent quotient score. *American Journal of Obstetrics and Gynecology* **128**, 486.

Tylden, E. (1973). The effects of maternal drug abuse on the foetus and the infant. *Adverse Drug Reaction Bulletin* **38**, 120.

Webster, P.A.C. (1973). Withdrawal symptoms in neonates associated with maternal antidepressant therapy. *Lancet* **2**, 318.

Weinstein, M.R. (1976). The international register of lithium babies. *Drug Information Journal* **2**, 94.

# 17

# Malignant disease in pregnancy

Maternal malignancy as a complication of pregnancy occurs once in every 1000–1500 pregnancies. Metastasis of a malignancy to the placenta and/or fetus is rare and less than 50 cases have been reported to date. Malignant melanoma is the commonest malignancy to involve the products of conception and accounts for a third of the cases. Haematopoietic malignancies (leukaemia and lymphoma) and breast carcinoma account for another third and the remaining third is distributed among various sarcomas and carcinomas. Fetal involvement is even rarer than placental involvement. Placental examination for metastatic deposits is important, as if it is involved, the likelihood of metastatic disease in the fetus is high.

## Carcinoma of the breast

The incidence of carcinoma of the breast in pregnancy is about 2 in 10 000 pregnancies and it becomes more common as maternal age increases. If the patient presents with a palpable tumour it is likely to exceed 1 cm in diameter and in the pregnant patient may be difficult to detect because of the breast changes associated with pregnancy.

### Investigation

It has been suggested that the routine thermographic, xeroradiographic or mammographic screening of the breasts of pregnant women over 25 years old may result in the earlier detection of tumours. Women with a family history of breast cancer are at an increased risk of developing the disease.

### Treatment

The treatment should be no different from the non-pregnant state. Pregnancy is not a contraindication to radical surgery and even radiotherapy may be undertaken without adverse effect on the fetus. Therapeutic abortion does not appear to influence the course of the disease favourably. About a third of women in whom breast cancer is diagnosed during pregnancy survive 5 years, but if detected early the figure rises to 60 per cent.

# Carcinoma of the colon

About 8 per cent of colorectal cancers are diagnosed before the age of 40 years, but only 200 cases associated with pregnancy have been reported and the incidence is said to be 1 in 100 000 pregnancies (McLean *et al*, 1955). The majority of the cancers are rectal, but the diagnosis is not usually made until the second trimester and is often associated with extensive metastatic deposits.

## Investigation

Although cancer of the colon is a rare complication of pregnancy it should be included in the differential diagnosis of a patient with colonic symptoms. The presence of rectal bleeding, abdominal pain, changing bowel habits, weight loss, palpable abdominal mass or persistent nausea and vomiting in late pregnancy should alert the clinician to the possibility of carcinoma of the colon. Sigmoidoscopy and colonoscopy must be considered.

## Treatment

If early diagnosis is made during pregnancy the appropriate surgery should be carried out forthwith. An early pregnancy may have to be terminated while in late pregnancy delivery of the baby by Caesarian section at the time of the definitive operation may be appropriate. The maternal prognosis is poor and 8 of the 18 patients described by Green *et al*, (1975) died within 3 months of diagnosis.

# Renal carcinoma

The most common presenting symptom in 17 pregnant women with renal cell carcinoma was a palpable mass (*Ney et al*, 1971). Only half had haematuria, a much lower percentage than the usual 75 per cent seen in non-pregnant women. Fever was seen in only three patients. The symptoms and signs of renal carcinoma in pregnancy are such that the patient is likely to present late with an unfavourable prognosis. Surgical removal is the treatment of choice.

# Carcinoma of the bladder

This is usually a disease of old age and is often associated with exposure to chemical carcinogens such as anilene dyes. It is consequently unusual to see it during pregnancy. However, in areas where schistosmiasis is common, bladder cancer may occur during the child bearing period. If it is detected early in pregnancy, anterior pelvic exenteration should be undertaken immediately. In late pregnancy, Caesarian section followed by anterior exenteration either immediately or at an interval of 10–14 days will save the fetus and decrease uterine size and pelvic vascularity.

# Ovarian carcinoma

Malignant ovarian tumours are rarely found in pregnancy and less than two hundred cases have been reported. If the disease is in a very early stage (1a) unilateral removal of the ovary and adjacent organs may be undertaken and the pregnancy allowed to continue, provided that the pathology is of a pseudomucinous cystadenocarcinoma, dysgerminoma, granulosatheca cell tumour, arrhenoblastoma, gynandroblastoma or possibly a low grade papillary tumour. With more advanced or more malignant disease the pregnancy should be terminated and a total hysterectomy performed.

# Malignant melanoma

Most authors report little difference between the survival of pregnant and non-pregnant patients with early melanoma. However, when the disease is more advanced the prognosis is much poorer in pregnant women. There is also some evidence that advanced disease occurs with greater frequency in pregnant women. In view of these reports all suspicious lesions should be removed with wide excision of the surrounding skin.

# Hodgkin's disease

This condition may occur at any age, but is particularly common between 20 and 30 years old. Most commonly the disease presents with painless enlargement of lymph nodes. If mediastinal nodes are involved there may be obstruction of the superior vena cava causing cyanosis and distension of the veins of the neck and upper chest wall. Narrowing of the trachea and major bronchi may cause cough and dyspnoea. Pruritus is common and herpes zoster may occur when vertebrae are involved in the disease. Systemic manifestations can occur early and include fatigue, malaise, fever, sweats, pruritus, anorexia

**Table 17.1** Causes of lymph node enlargement which must be excluded in the diagnosis of Hodgkin's disease

| | |
|---|---|
| *Bacterial* | Acute bacterial infections |
| | Tuberculosis |
| *Viral* | Infectious mononucleosis |
| | Cytomegalovirus |
| *Other infections* | Toxoplasmosis |
| | Cat scratch fever |
| *Idiopathic* | Sarcoidosis |
| | Diseases with autoimmune features |

and weight loss. Constitutional upset infers widespread disease and indicates an unfavourable prognosis.

## Investigation

Firstly one must exclude some infective, inflammatory or chemical cause. The next step is to establish a tissue diagnosis by means of biopsy of an enlarged lymph node. The principal features differentiating Hodgkin's disease from non-Hodgkin's lymphoma are the presence of Sternberg–Reed giant cells with their characteristic prominent nucleoli and variable numbers of lymphoid cells.

The extent of the disease is usually assessed so that an appropriate plan of treatment may be developed. These usually include lower limb lymphangiography, chest X-ray, bone marrow aspiration and a staging laparotomy or CT scanning. Obviously in pregnancy such procedures are limited.

## Treatment

The occurrence of pregnancy does not alter the prognosis of Hodgkin's disease (Barry *et al*, 1962), but it may affect the extent of investigation. In patients with Hodgkin's disease who become pregnant, the main problem is in those who continue chemotherapy for relatively advanced disease. Therapeutic abortion may be considered because of the hazard of teratogenicity and fetal abnormality. However, many patients are on relatively safe drugs such as steroids and azathioprine and each case has to be judged on its merits.

The following guidelines have been suggested (Kaplan, 1972).

1. Localized disease diagnosed at 30 weeks gestation or later should have minimal diagnostic or therapeutic intervention until after delivery, which should be as early as possible.
2. Advanced disease in late pregnancy is treated conservatively with single drug chemotherapy aimed at palliation and successful completion of the pregnancy.

3. Diagnosis before 20 weeks may warrant therapeutic termination and a subsequent laparotomy for fixation of the ovaries in the midline prior to irradiation (Peckham and McElwain, 1973).

The use of radiotherapy for localized disease may be considered during pregnancy and has been undertaken without danger to the fetus (Kaplan, 1972).

# References

Garry, R.M., Diamond, H.D. and Craver, L.F. (1962). Influence of pregnancy on course of Hodgkin's disease. *American Journal of Obstetrics and Gynecology* **84**, 445.

Green, L.K., Harris, R.E. and Massey, F.M. (1975). Cancer of the colon during pregnancy. *Obstetrics and Gynecology* **46**, 480.

Kaplan, H.S. (1972). *Hodgkin's Disease*. Harvard University Press, Massachussetts.

Karim, M., Ammar, R. and Dadawy, S. (1968). Carcinoma of the bladder with pregnancy. *Journal of the Egyptian Medical Association* **51**, 1037–52.

McLean, D.W., Arminski, T.C. and Bradley, G.T. (1955). Management of primary carcinoma of the rectum during pregnancy. *American Journal of Surgery* **90**, 816.

Ney, C., Posner, A.C. and Ehrlich, J.C. (1971). Tubular adenoma of the kidney during pregnancy. *Obstetrics and Gynecology* **37**, pp. 267–76.

Peckham, M.J. and McElwain, T.J. (1973). *Hodgkin's Disease*. Edited by Smithers. D. Churchill Livingstone, Edinburgh.

Pelosi, M., Hung, C.T., Langer, A., Khademi, M. and Harrigan, J.T. (1975). Renal carcinoma in pregnancy. *Obstetrics and Gynecology* **45**, 461.

Riberti, C., Marola, G. and Bertani, A. (1981). Malignant melanoma: the adverse effect of pregnancy. *British Journal of Plastic Surgery* **34**, 338.

Torres, J.E. and Mickal, A. (1975). Carcinoma of the breast in pregnancy. *Clinical Obstetrics and Gynecology* **18**, 219.

Yamasaki, M. *et al*. (1975). Malignant ovarian tumours in pregnancy. *Acta Obstetrica Gynaecologica Japonica* **22**, 138.

# 18

# Normal results in pregnancy

**Table 18.1** Normal results in pregnancy

**Haematology**

| | Trimester First | Second | Third |
|---|---|---|---|
| White cell count (× 10⁹/litre) | 5–12 | 6–15 | 6–14 |
| Red cell count (× 10¹²/litre) | 3.5–4.6 | 3.3–4.3 | 3.4–4.4 |
| Haemoglobin (g/dl) | 10.8–13.2 | 10.5–12.9 | 10.6–13.8 |
| Haematocrit (%) | 31–39 | 30–38 | 32–40 |
| Mean corpuscular volume (fl) | 80–94 | 84–98 | 84–98 |
| Mean corpuscular haemoglobin (pg) | 27.5–31.5 | 28.5–32.5 | 28.5–32.5 |
| Mean corpuscular haemoglobin concentration (g/dl) | 32–36 | 32–36 | 32–36 |
| Serum ferritin (micrograms/litre) | 30 | 10 | 6 |
| Serum folate (micrograms/litre) | 3–10 } | Both values fall as pregnancy | |
| Red cell folate (micrograms/litre) | 120–350 } | advances | |
| Serum iron ($\mu$mol/litre) | 10.7–21.4 | There are variations in this value throughout the day with the highest measurement being in the morning | |
| Total iron binding capacity ($\mu$mol/litre) | 50–80 | | |
| Vitamin $B_{12}$ (ng/litre) | 200–350 | This level falls throughout pregnancy | |

*Biochemistry*

| | | | |
|---|---|---|---|
| Plasma cortisol (nmol/litre) | 552–1104 | 552–1104 | This level increases during the last trimester |

*Thyroid function*

| | | | |
|---|---|---|---|
| Serum triiodothyronine (nmol/litre) | 1.9–4.3 | 2.2–4.8 | 2.2–4.3 |
| Serum thyroxine (nmol/litre) | 89–217 | 100–228 | 96–227 |
| Thyroid stimulating hormone (mU/litre) | 2.9 | 2.6 | 2.1 |

*Blood glucose*

| | | | |
|---|---|---|---|
| Fasting venous sample (mmol/litre) | >5 is abnormal and indicative of diabetes | | |
| Glycosylated haemoglobin (%) | 5.5–9.5 | These values are reduced from 20 weeks | |

**Table 18.1** Normal results in pregnancy

**Haematology**

| | Trimester First | Second | Third |
|---|---|---|---|
| *Hepatic function* | | | |
| Bilirubin (μmol/litre) | 2–14 | 2–14 | 2–14 |
| Alkaline phosphatase (i.u/litre) | 20–150 | This level increases from the fifth week to term | |
| Cholesterol (mmol/litre) | 4–11 | The levels are raised throughout pregnancy | |
| Total protein (g/dl) | 6–8 | There is a fall to 85 % of these values during the first trimester and then the levels are constant | |
| Albumin (g/dl) | 3.8–4.6 | 3.3–4.4 | 2.5–4.1 |
| Globulins | $\alpha$ and $\beta$ fractions increase and $\gamma$ globulins show a small fall | | |
| *Renal function* | | | |
| Urea (mmol/l) | Values above 4.5 mmol/l are abnormal | | |
| Serum creatinine (μmol/litre) | 60–70 | 46–56 | 64–74 |

# 19

# Drugs in pregnancy and during breast feeding

## Drugs in pregnancy

In general, the harmful effects of drugs during pregnancy cause congenital malformations in the first trimester and in subsequent trimesters impair growth and function. Drugs given prior to delivery may have an effect on the neonate after birth.

**Table 19.1** Common drugs and their use in pregnancy

| Drug group | Use and associated problems |
|---|---|
| **Cardiovascular drugs** | |
| Diuretics | These drugs should not be used to treat hypertension in pregnancy as they cause reduced plasma volume and placental perfusion |
| β blockers | These drugs are useful for the treatment of hypertension but may cause neonatal hypoglycaemia and bradycardia |
| Heparin | Prolonged useage can result in maternal osteoporosis |
| Oral anticoagulants | Warfarin is preferred to phenindione |
| **Respiratory drugs** | |
| Aminophylline | Neonatal irritability has been reported |
| **Endocrine drugs** | |
| Carbimazole | Neonatal goitre and hypothyroidism can result from its administration to the pregnant woman |
| Corticosteroids | Doses greater than 10 mg of prednisolone daily may lead to fetal adrenal suppression |
| **Neurological drugs** | |
| Phenytoin and phenobarbitone | These drugs may cause congenital malformations. However, the risk of untreated epilepsy to the fetus is uncertain. The neonate may have a bleeding tendency |
| Sodium valproate | This drug may cause neural tube defects in the fetus |
| **Psychiatric drugs** | |
| Alcohol | This can cause the fetal alcohol syndrome |
| Benzodiazepines | These drugs may cause neonatal drowsiness and the floppy baby syndrome |

**Table 19.1** Common drugs and their use in pregnancy

| Drug group | Use and associated problems |
| --- | --- |
| Lithium | Congenital malformations and neonatal goitre may result |
| **Antibiotics** | |
| Aminoglycosides | Auditory or vestibular nerve damage may occur in the fetus |
| Chloramphenicol | This drug can cause the grey baby syndrome |
| Sulphonamides | These drugs can precipitate neonatal kernicterus |
| Tetracyclines | This drug may cause acute fatty liver in the mother and neonatal dental discolouration |

# Self-poisoning with common 'over the counter' drugs

Both aspirin and paracetamol (acetaminophen) are commonly used in attempted self-poisoning. Psychological support is a particularly important aspect of the management of such incidents in pregnancy. However, both aspirin and paracetamol overdoses can be fatal and require active medical management.

# Aspirin

Early toxic symptoms of aspirin overdose include vertigo, tinnitus and impaired hearing. Hyperpnoea may be an early symptom of serious poisoning. Nausea, vomiting, drowsiness, visual impairment, confusion, hallucinations, fitting and coma may follow.

## Investigation

Blood salicylates are of value. Serious poisoning in the non-pregnant adult is rare at levels less than 50 mg/100 ml. Levels greater than 100 mg/100 ml during the first 6 hours after the overdose indicate severe poisoning and may be fatal. During pregnancy salicylate is readily transferred from mother to fetus across the placenta. The fetus eliminates salicylate slowly because of immature glucuronidation and renal excretion. Consequently it accumulates in the fetus and is present for longer periods and in higher doses than in the mother. Its volume of distribution is also greater in the fetus near term and in the newborn child than in older children and adults. Consequently a given plasma level of aspirin in the newborn reflects a larger amount of drug per unit of body weight than in older children.

## Treatment

In view of the differential accumulation of aspirin in the fetus, treatment should begin at lower maternal plasma levels (e.g. 30 mg/100 ml). Treatment is largely supportive and gastric lavage should be considered. Electrolyte disturbances can be corrected with the appropriate intravenous solutions but a forced alkaline diuresis is hazardous and should not be undertaken. Haemodialysis is very effective for the removal of salicylates from seriously poisoned patients.

There are few published reports of the effect of aspirin self-poisoning on the outcome of pregnancy. It has been suggested that fetal death can result, although a number of pregnancies have reached term successfully. A high aspirin level at the end of a pregnancy may result in maternal and fetal haemorrhage.

# Paracetamol (Acetaminophen)

Self-poisoning with paracetamol can cause massive hepatic necrosis and this effect is dose dependent and exacerbated by alcohol; a quantity as small as 15 g may be fatal. After an initial period of anorexia, nausea and vomiting, the patient may appear well for 2 or 3 days. Subsequently liver failure can develop.

Studies on fetal hepatic cells have shown a reduced ability to neutralize paracetamol metabolites by forming glucuronide and sulphate conjugates. Once these conjugation pathways are depleted toxic metabolites accumulate and covalently bind with tissue macromolecules and cause hepatic necrosis.

## Investigation

Plasma paracetamol levels should be measured. If they are above a line plotted between 300 mg/litre at 4 hours and 45 mg/litre at 15 hours there is a high risk of hepatic necrosis. Concentrations below this level but above a 'treatment line' between 200 mg/litre at 4 hours and 30 mg/litre at 15 hours are at intermediate risk and will have significant benefit from an infusion of intravenous N-acetyl cysteine.

## Treatment

Acetyl cysteine may protect the liver by restoring depleted glutathione or by acting as an alternative substrate for paracetamol metabolites. 150 mg/kg body weight should be infused over 15 minutes in 200 ml of 5 % dextrose followed by an infusion of 50 mg/kg body weight in 500 ml of 5 % dextrose over the next 4 hours and 100 mg/kg body weight over the following 16 hours. Acetyl cysteine is effective if given during the first 8 hours after an overdose but is subsequently of less value and may be harmful 15 hours after ingestion of paracetamol. Its safety in pregnancy is unknown and it may, or may not, cross the placenta. It has been given in the second and third trimesters without apparent adverse effects.

## Drugs in breast milk

The interpretation of the literature about drugs and breast feeding has three main difficulties. Often there is no relevant information available for the drug. When information is available, it is often poor in quality and even when it is of good quality, it is often omitted from review articles and data sheets.

Toxicity to the infant can occur if the drug enters breast milk in sufficient quantities. This is seen with iodides, benzodiazepines such as diazepam and barbiturates.

**Table 19.2** Drugs in breast milk

| Drug group | Adverse effects on infant reported | Relatively safe drugs |
|---|---|---|
| *Analgesics and anti-inflammatory drugs* | Gold<br>Indomethacin<br>Phenylbutazone | Codeine<br>Ibuprofen<br>Mefenamic Acid<br>Paracetamol<br>Pethidine<br>Salicylates |
| *Antibiotics* | Aminoglycosides<br>Chloramphenicol | Antifungals<br>Cephalosporins<br>Erythromycin<br>Penicillins |
| *Anticoagulants* | Phenindione | Heparin<br>Warfarin |
| *Antihypertensives and cardiac drugs* | Amiodarone | $\beta$ blockers<br>Hydrallazine<br>Digoxin |
| *Neurological drugs* | Lithium<br>Alcohol | Benzodiazepines<br>Phenothiazines<br>Sodium valproate<br>Tricyclics |
| *Endocrine drugs* | Oestrogens<br>Carbimazole | Steroids<br>Insulin<br>Progestogens |

# Further reading

*British National Formulary*. British Medical Association and the Pharmaceutical Society of Great Britain.

Beeley, L. (1983). *Safer Prescribing. A Guide To Some Problems In The Use Of Drugs*. Blackwell Scientific Publications, Oxford.

# Index

# Index